THE MOTHER EARTH EFFECT

CONNECT TO THE EARTH AND HEAL

ELISABETH HOEKSTRA

OLIVIA RAMIREZ SMITH

First Edition

Library of Congress Control Number: 2022921015

ISBN: 979-8-9871224-0-2

Publisher info:

4biddenknowledge Inc

business@4biddenknowledge.com

Cover art and Epigraph by Taya Crayk-Bonde

Cover design by Laura C. Cantu, @LauraCCantu

Interior design by Christine Contini, Winterwolf Press

DEDICATION

With gratitude, we dedicate this book to the women who gathered to share their recovery stories so that any sisters in need may learn about and experience the therapeutic health benefits naturally received when grounding their bodies with Mother Earth's subtle healing energies.

OUR MOTHER
BY TAYA CRAYK-BONDE

" I am the mother to all.
I give the breath to your lungs,
I give the magic to the seed which makes it grow,
I am the wonder that no one can explain.
I am part of everything you create.
You are a part of me,
just as I am a part of you.
I am intricately woven with the universe,
the stars, the moon, the sun.
I am the rush of the ocean waves,
I am the breeze that gently tussles your hair,
I am the billowing clouds dancing gracefully in
the sky,
I carry the warm rays that kiss your face,
I am the water that quenches all thirst,
I am the food that provides all life.
I am a billion different species,
creating the experience called life.
I am the beauty that feeds your soul,
not just your eyes.
No one truly owns parts of me,
For I belong to everyone equally.
I am the one true home for every being,
From before,
The here and now,
For the rest of eternity."

- Mother Earth

REVIEWS

"The Mother Earth Effect is a wonderful account of why connecting to the earth is critical to our health and well-being. Grounding is essential in my life and, it's one of the most important things I do on a daily(and nightly) basis"
Mariel Hemingway
Actress/Writer/Speaker
Runs MH Foundation for mental health

"The Mother Earth Effect is an intriguing book on the healing powers of earthing. It is filled with fascinating stories and ways to use this technology that can help you in your daily lives. I recommend it."
Daniel G. Amen, MD
Founder of Amen Clinics
Author of Change Your Brain Every Day

"The Mother Earth Effect is a mind blowing book with real-life stories that will pull at your heartstrings. Great inspiration for all ages. This book is MUST READ!"
Billy Carson, Two times Best Selling Author of
Compendium Of The Emerald Tablets

and Woke Doesn't Mean Broke
4biddenknowledge.com

"The book is well-written, easy to read, and to understand. The stories are amazing and very compelling! What I like the most is the matter-of-fact approach focused on the importance of having an open mind and trying earthing. I too was skeptical. I just kept an open mind to experience it. The benefits were unmistakable. I hope readers get enticed to try earthing after reading this book."
Gaétan Chevalier, Ph.D.
Director, Earthing Institute

"It was Elisabeth who introduced me to Grounding. A simple word between friends during a conversation. Since then, the view of my body and the world around me has fundamentally changed. 'The Mother Earth Effect' is a work that will do the same for you- get ready, you are about to transform the micro to the macro… all of it."
Jimmy Church
Radio, TV, and Film Host
FADE to BLACK

"The Mother Earth Effect" is a MUST-READ for all walks of life. These life-changing stories will leave you amazed, inspired, intrigued, and wanting to experience grounding for yourself. Each woman's heartfelt story compiled in this book is a true testament that proves connecting to the source, Mother Earth, can help with so many different ailments. In chiropractic, we educate our patients that inflammation is the root of all diseases. Through my own experience, I have become a huge advocate for grounding. This practice has proven to decrease inflammation decrease pain, improve the quality of sleep and bring a sense of calm to your mind, body, and soul."
Andréa Mosca, Doctor of Chiropractic
NREMT - ICU Medical Technician
Podcast host of Dr.Dré Your Health Bae

"The Mother Earth Effect introduces readers to the health, natural healing energies, and power of grounding. It's an eye-opening book that shows us how we've disconnected from the Earth and how to easily reconnect and enjoy the many potential benefits. For me, walking barefoot in nature reduces my stress and provides clarity. A must-read if you want to learn simple ways to reconnect with the ground beneath your feet and rebalance."

Lisa Vrancken
#1 bestselling author of Sacred Spaces
BE...From Passion and Purpose to Product and Prosperity
Award-winning TV Producer

"The stories in this book will inspire you to kick your shoes off and reunite with the earth, equip your bed with a grounding mat and shout the phenomenal benefits of grounding from the rooftops! There is nothing better to demonstrate our energetic connection to nature than the miracle of these real-life stories!"

Dr. Sheila Lewis Ealey & Sumayyah Simone
MyBlackHealth.com

"*The Mother Earth Effect* is a great introduction to the world of reducing inflammation and biological stress. While most people are running around discussing the problem, Elisabeth and Olivia are giving powerful solutions that can be applied to so many issues. Plus, explaining our interconnection with this powerful effect can elevate your spiritual awareness. I recommend you read and share this message with all those you love."

Patrick K. Porter, PhD Founder & Inventor of BrainTap®
The Brain Fitness Company™

CONTENTS

FOREWORD

Nearly thirty years ago, an ethereal blue image of a woman appeared before me in a dream. This beautiful woman carried a powerful, quiet presence. I remember that she looked at me sternly and, speaking with her eyes alone, said, "We are waiting for you." To do what, there was no clue.

About a year later, with little more than a faint memory of the first dream, I experienced a similar dream. This time I saw a close-up of the woman's eyes. As her image began to fade, I saw in her eyes an expression of her concern.

As the years went on, I had several similar dreams, all with faint silhouettes of women's eyes staring at me. Each new dream prompted memories of the earlier ones, but like all the others, they quickly faded away.

It was in the late 1990s that I became interested in researching the health effects of people losing their ground when wearing non-conductive plastic-soled shoes. To most, this would seem an odd thing to investigate. Except for me, a person with a thirty-year background in grounding electrical equipment, it made complete sense.

Shortly after publishing my original grounding research and with the dreams still a mystery, I had another dream. This time the women's eyes grimaced with pain. Then, came more dreams in a short period, all of the women with eyes in pain. But like all the dreams that came before, even these soon faded away.

To begin the earthing studies, we created straightforward ways to ground subjects' bodies to the earth. The first method was an EKG patch attached to a subject's body and to the earth via an electrical outlet ground. For the sleep studies, we created conductive carbon mats to place on subjects' beds for overnight and long-term monitoring.

The benefit subjects reported most from grounding was instant pain reduction. The second was improved sleep. As a result, nearly all test subjects and even the researchers asked if they could keep the study mats, and many asked if we had any extras they could take home for their moms or other family members. With each new study, the demand for patches and mats continued to grow.

My last dream with the familiar ethereal blue silhouette of a woman was about twelve years ago. The final dream that came was different. She was lying on a pillow with her eyes closed, peacefully sleeping. I instantly woke from the dream with a complete realization of the connection between the women in my dreams and the earthing research.

This book contains the rest of the story!

Thank you, Elisabeth, and Olivia, for bringing these women's stories to light.

—Clint

INTRODUCTION

Beneath your feet lies an amazing gift from Nature with the potential to quickly restore your health, balance, and quality of life. This gift is the very Earth we live on. Earth is naturally equipped with a surprisingly built-in healing power that may be the most effective medicine available.

Earthing, also known as grounding, is a major discovery showing that contact with this natural energy stabilizes the way the body works at the deepest level, draining it of inflammation, pain, and stress, and generating greater well-being.

Over many years after a seemingly innocuous shift in the design of shoes from leather to plastics and rubber, Electron-deficit disorders developed. Electron-deficit disorders refer to a wide variety of conditions that have quietly come to interfere with our wellness.

Modern research has documented disastrous shifts in our biology and health caused by a lack of contact with the surface of the Earth. Our modern lifestyles have separated us from nature's best antioxidants and from important biological rhythms.

Fortunately, these shifts are easily remedied with the practice of Earthing. This discovery represents a health and healing breakthrough and has been creating a big buzz in the health world since the release of the Earthing study and book.

Earthing is accessible to everyone and is as simple as walking or sitting barefoot outdoors on the ground or laying on the ground with skin contact on the earth. At any moment that you have pain, go out and try it. Your connection to Earth will knock down and knock out inflammation in your body. That's an effect with massive benefits.

Inflammation is considered a primary cause or aggravator of chronic and aging-related disorders. These disorders include:

- cardiovascular diseases
- diabetes
- arthritis
- autoimmune disorders
- Alzheimer's
- cancer
- depression
- autism

Inflammation is like having a silent fire inside your body. Earthing restores a lost electric connection to the Earth. People feel, sleep, and look better, as a result. They have more energy and vitality. Earthing is a natural healing strategy that works for all ages, from the youngest to the oldest.

Earthing reconnects you to an abandoned aspect of Nature— Mother Earth's healing touch. Due to the overwhelming demand by participants in the Earthing research study, Earthing was born. Earthing offers a multitude of products that connect your body to the natural healing energy of the earth when indoors while sleeping, relaxing, or working. This is a great option for those who are unable to earth outside due to weather or for those who want to maximize their time connecting to the Earth.

THE MOTHER EARTH EFFECT

CIRCULATION, PAIN, & INFLAMMATION

OLIVIA RAMIREZ SMITH

"*W*hat are you going to do with these cords?"

I stood in the exhibit center of the medical conference in Los Angeles and watched an elderly gentleman on his knees place coil cords with grounding patches under a row of chairs.

"They are for people to ground themselves."

While still on his knees, Clint looked at me and pointed to some screens.

"We can see with thermographic images the decrease of inflammation in their bodies after grounding for thirty minutes. Lower levels of inflammation produce a reduction in pain."

His matter-a-fact words left me with a blank stare. Everything he said other than *a reduction in pain* made no sense.

Fortunately, he stood up and took another approach.

"Do you have any pain?"

"Yes, maybe a little." I didn't share that I had chronic pain in my leg from poor circulation; nothing ever helped my constant discomfort.

Clint gestured to a chair, "Sit down. It will be easier to show you rather than try to explain it."

I sat down, and he placed patches on the bottom of each of my feet. He connected the patches to the coil cords.

"What are the cords connected to?" I asked, my head tilting sideways as I looked to follow the cord.

"To a ground rod driven into the earth."

The idea struck me as completely bizarre, but since I was already patched up, I decided to give it a go. In less than ten minutes, the chronic pain in my left leg and the bottom of my feet magically drained away. My toes, colored purple from the poor circulation, returned to the typical color of healthy skin.

I sat there in disbelief.

How was it possible that in less than ten minutes, my pain was gone, and the circulation in my feet returned to normal? Whatever magic this was, I needed to know more. Heck, I wanted to grab it and take it home. Every one of my chronic pain clients needed whatever this was.

That night, I read straight through the paperback copy I picked up of the gentleman's book called *Earthing*. I could not put it down.

It turns out that grounding the body to the earth, like standing barefoot in the backyard, naturally reduces inflammation and pain. The pain lessens as the ground equalizes the electrical charges between the body and the Earth.

Even though the information astounded me, had I not experienced the instant pain relief earlier that day, I doubt I would have believed what I read. The idea that Mother Earth profoundly and directly affects our health surprised me.

In 2012, I went to this conference on a mission to find effective treatments for our spa client's many physical disorders. I wanted to help them recover and get their lives back. Something so simple that every one of my patrons could benefit from using.

I left the conference with the Holy Grail.

Eager to get this health revolution started, I hooked my family up with the sample pillowcases Clint gave at the conference.

The first night on the grounded pillowcase, I fell into a deep coma-like sleep and woke rested and refreshed—something not experienced by me in years.

At work, I eagerly shared my miraculous findings. Most of my staff just rolled their eyes and gave me a look. I needed more support than just some skeptical and dismissive looks.

Immediately, I contacted the research people who made the mats and pillowcases and ordered a dozen of each. I then scheduled a weekend event at our spa and invited the entire town to experience the healing effect of grounding for free.

During the event, we grounded dozens of clients using mats and patches. The results were unreal! Those who experienced the thirty-minute session reported instant relief from chronic foot, knee, and joint pain.

However, the show stopper that grabbed all the attention was how much younger and healthier everyone looked after grounding. They all marveled at the increased energy they received and left feeling better than when they arrived.

One year later, I sold my spa. With a new mission in mind, *I implemented a plan to have women remove their shoes and experience the Mother Earth Effect!*[1]

----

1. Research References
    9. Classification of EEG Signal for Body Earthing Application 2018
    https://earthinginstitute.net/wp-content/uploads/2021/10/RahmanAl.EEG_for_Body-Earthing_Application-2018-1.pdf
    14. One-Hour Contact with the Earth's Surface (Grounding) Improves Inflammation and Blood Flow—A Randomized, Double-Blind, Pilot Study 2015
    www.scirp.org/Journal/PaperInformation.aspx?PaperID=58836
    15The Effect of Grounding the Human Body on Mood 2015
    prx.sagepub.com/content/116/2/534.full.pdf+html
    22. Emotional Stress, Heart Rate Variability, Grounding, and Improved Autonomic Tone: Clinical Applications 2011
    https://earthinginstitute.net/wp-content/uploads/2016/07/Emotional-stress-study.pdf
    30. The Biologic Effects of Grounding the Human Body During Sleep as

Measured by Cortisol Levels and Subjective Reporting of Sleep, Pain, and Stress 2004
   https://earthinginstitute.net/wp-content/uploads/2016/07/Cortisol-Study.pdf
   42. Earthing: health implications of reconnecting the human body to the Earth's surface electrons.
   https://pubmed.ncbi.nlm.nih.gov/22291721/
   46. The effect of grounding the human body on mood.
   https://pubmed.ncbi.nlm.nih.gov/25748085/
   52. The biologic effects of grounding the human body during sleep as measured by cortisol levels and subjective reporting of sleep, pain, and stress.
   https://pubmed.ncbi.nlm.nih.gov/15650465/

JUST LIKE CHRISTMAS

DIAPHRAGMATIC BREATH, REDUCTION IN STRESS, & CALM

ELISABETH HOEKSTRA

*W*henever I receive a new bio-hacking tool in the mail, it feels like Christmas. I'm like a kid at a candy store, and the true nerd that I am comes out.

Like with my silver-threaded sheet I found on Amazon. When I first put my purchase on my bed, it helped me sleep through the night without waking up. This difference lasted about a month before my nighttime behavior returned to normal, meaning I woke up every night around 3-4 AM with slight trouble falling back asleep. I figured the product needed to be replaced because something went wrong.

I set out to surf the Internet as I do, to keep up to date with the latest technology in the bio-hacking field. During this search for a replacement, an ad from a company called "Earthing" popped up with a Father's Day special. This sales pitch reminded me of my solid nights of sleep, which straight away sold me on the products.

I chose a package with a bed sheet, a pillowcase, and those patches that you can stick anywhere on your body—what a great deal.

The box arrived on my doorstep within a week, and it was Christmas again.

I ripped it open and dumped out the contents. Everyone who's met me knows that I do not half-ass anything. I go all the way in. True to form, I placed the sheet on my bed, pillowcase on my pillow, and a patch on my solar plexus and connected them all to the ground in my outlets. I lay flat on my back on my bed, skin to the mat, and closed my eyes to go into my body and feel whatever happened next.

To my complete astonishment, five minutes after laying down and immersing myself in the grounding items, I felt a sense of calm. In my thirty-one years of life, I had never experienced such a quick and easy connection to relaxation.

At this point, I knew something was unique about this purchase. This company specialized specifically in the science of Earthing, and as I learned during my research, the CEO is the man that rediscovered this healing modality in the late 1990s. Unlike the silver threaded bed cover I got from Amazon, this sheet and pillowcase were 100% carbon and had a lifetime warranty, guaranteed to be long-lasting.

I lay engulfed in the calm sensation and continued to go into my body to feel this profound alteration. Only a few minutes after lying down, I took a different breath, a breath that went deeper and deeper past my stomach, past my belly button, and almost down to my pelvic floor.

I lay astonished at the moment, not only because of my twenty years as a cigarette smoker but because I had never taken such a breath. I felt utterly alive for the first time. This extraordinary shift in my body brought me almost to tears. Before this, like most people, my breath stayed high in my chest. With each consecutive and deepening abdominal breath, my excitement grew.

My breath gave life to a new obsession!

This modality altered my life forever.

FROM THAT POINT, I dove deep into the research behind this life-changing discovery. I watched The Earthing Movie and read the book that came with the products. In addition, I continuously grounded and devoured every case study I could get my hands on. Because of the profound and extravagant positive changes from practicing this phenomenon, I couldn't digest enough information about it. I wanted to know everything...

Whenever possible, I go to the origin of a source to find the most facts I can. My starvation for knowledge pushed me. I must have at least one conversation with the man who created these Earthing products.

I found him on LinkedIn. Not expecting any response, I kept my fingers crossed and shot him a message. Days later, a note appeared in my inbox, which led me to my face-to-face meet and greet with the man himself, Clint Ober.

My heart raced as I watched Clint walk into the small meeting room where I and others waited. A beautiful woman named Olivia followed close behind him. I felt her energy as soon as she stepped into the room. This soft, sweet, assertive, and feisty short, dark-haired woman sat next to Clint.

I introduced myself and my team. At the time, I held the position of President at a mental health and trauma facility. Shortly after our quick introductions, we heard from Brisa Alfaro. She was a friend of my associates and a stroke survivor. We brought her along to test out Earthing.

That day, a miracle happened right in front of my eyes. This life-changing meeting affected us all, and we gobbled up every bit of this master's grounding knowledge he offered.

For me, the evidence sparked a fire, a desire to scream the benefits of this healing technique to anyone who would hear me.

Life forever changed.[1]

---

1. Research References
9. Classification of EEG Signal for Body Earthing Application 2018
https://earthinginstitute.net/wp-content/uploads/2021/10/RahmanAl.EEG_for_Body-Earthing_Application-2018-1.pdf

14. One-Hour Contact with the Earth's Surface (Grounding) Improves Inflammation and Blood Flow—A Randomized, Double-Blind, Pilot Study 2015
www.scirp.org/Journal/PaperInformation.aspx?PaperID=58836
15The Effect of Grounding the Human Body on Mood 2015
prx.sagepub.com/content/116/2/534.full.pdf+html
22. Emotional Stress, Heart Rate Variability, Grounding, and Improved Autonomic Tone: Clinical Applications 2011
https://earthinginstitute.net/wp-content/uploads/2016/07/Emotional-stress-study.pdf
30. The Biologic Effects of Grounding the Human Body During Sleep as Measured by Cortisol Levels and Subjective Reporting of Sleep, Pain, and Stress 2004
https://earthinginstitute.net/wp-content/uploads/2016/07/Cortisol-Study.pdf
42. Earthing: health implications of reconnecting the human body to the Earth's surface electrons.
https://pubmed.ncbi.nlm.nih.gov/22291721/
46. The effect of grounding the human body on mood.
https://pubmed.ncbi.nlm.nih.gov/25748085/
52. The biologic effects of grounding the human body during sleep as measured by cortisol levels and subjective reporting of sleep, pain, and stress.
https://pubmed.ncbi.nlm.nih.gov/15650465/

3

THE GIFT OF GABBING

LOCKED-IN SYNDROME & PONS STROKE

BRISA ALFARO

*F*inding the strength to live has become my constant effort. Not too long ago, I lay motionless in a hospital bed because of a Pons Stroke. My body refused to respond to treatments, so I received a tracheotomy, which allowed machines to breathe for me.

When the time came to take out the breathing tube, the removal created scar tissue that reduced my air passage to the width of a straw. Terrified, I feared permanent damage to my airway.

Mercifully, scar tissue removal surgery helped me breathe again.

Regrettably, the difficulty returned. I struggled to breathe, eat, exercise, or just do life.

My scar tissue removal changed from a one-time experience to a reoccurring surgery every 6-9 months post-stroke. The repetition made me a pro. My post-surgery recovery included losing my speaking ability for three weeks and a no-solid food diet as it irritated my still raw airway. I learned to avoid things that increased my needed recovery time and physically made my body weaker. To keep from trying to whisper, as that gave me more pain and physically prolonged my healing, I spent my time writing on a whiteboard to communicate.

Following my latest surgery, with only two weeks of my recovery completed, I found myself in a meeting with Elisabeth Hoekstra, sitting across from Clint Ober. The group convinced me that this meeting came with life-changing possibilities.

My typical whiteboard communication strategy would not do. Instead, I sat ready to whisper with all my might. My heart raced, and before I began to speak, I noticed a cold sweat rise from my palms.

How would I be able to get my story out under these conditions?

On a mission, I started, my voice barely a harsh whisper.

Even though I knew very little about Clint's work with Earthing, I agreed to try anything to help the side effects that persisted following my stroke.

I remained open to all possibilities.

Three minutes into my whispering, Clint politely interrupted my very difficult-to-hear speech and asked to put a grounding patch on the palm of my hand.

Concerned about what the patch might do, he assured me the patch wouldn't hurt.

I agreed and watched as Clint snapped one side of a tiny red cord onto a medical lead and the other end of the cord to a plug, which he inserted into a wall socket. The plug stood as unique in the sense that it only had one prong for the metal ground.

Clint opened my hand and placed the patch on my exposed palm. I studied the snap button on the pad. I followed the small red cord back to the funny-looking plug that connected to the wall.

I waited in anticipation; I expected to feel something, but nothing happened.

"Please, continue," Clint encouraged.

I continued to share the details of the most profound days of my life. Following the Pons Stroke, I developed locked-in syndrome. Eight years before this day, I was literally trapped in my body, fully conscious. I could hear and see everything around me, but I couldn't move or speak.

With fewer than 5 cases per year worldwide, the doctors gave me less than 1% odds of recovery.

As I told my story, I traveled back and heard the doctors tell my mother, "There is no hope."

The emotions I encountered as they encouraged her to contact my family for their goodbyes returned. I relived the experience, and my eyes welled up with tears of gratitude for my family's strong support during that time. The plan my mother devised, regardless of what my medical report read, saved my life.

While I continued to talk about my journey to recovery, I noticed I became warm. A slight tingling sensation moved throughout my body.

Focused on my sharing, I disregarded the sensations until the startled looks my audience gave rendered me speechless.

These looks came from everyone in the room.

"Is everything okay?" I asked.

One of the attendees responded with a question of their own, "How do you feel?"

Everyone quietly waited, their attention focused on my neck.

Elisabeth Hoekstra exclaimed, "Look at her neck, look at her neck, there's a perfect circle there!"

Olivia, an affiliate of Clint and Ground Therapy, spoke up, "It's red there because the blood is going to that spot and nourishing the area of her surgery."

Could I be healing? I thought.

To my surprise, I realized my voice while sharing increased slowly from a soft, difficult whisper to a low, effortless tone. I experienced a never-before-felt change, and I had an audience to witness. Everyone in the room continued to stare at me in awe of what they saw and heard... everyone except for Clint.

Clint expected my change and sat completely without surprise. His calm demeanor gave me the comfort I needed. From the other side of the table, he smiled and shared, "Yes, things like this happen all of the time when I ground someone, please, continue with your story."

I continued, and with each minute that passed, I noticed greater ease in my ability to speak. I spoke with less effort, and the strength of my vocal cords appeared to be back!

As I wrapped up my share, I spoke in an almost *normal* tone!

Usually, after such a share, I am extremely exhausted from the effort. I found this time, I had more energy than I did before I walked into that room. I honestly didn't know what to think about the sudden change, but I did feel the trajectory of my life altered in some capacity.

Our lives changed; we all hugged it out and said our goodbyes.

Clint generously gifted me some grounding equipment to take home.

"YES!!" I was more than grateful to receive his gift of a conductive mattress pad, pillowcases, and some patches to take home along with his book, *Earthing*.

Prior to my stroke, I never in a million years would have thought that I could ever be this excited about discovering an improvement for my health. However, I left there that afternoon completely elated and ready to implement all my new tools!

ON THE WAY HOME, I looked at my companion, "I'm tired of eating mashed-up food, I just want to chew! Let's stop somewhere to eat real food. I think I'm ready!"

Even though my latest surgery occurred two weeks ago, my voice sounded significantly stronger. The recovery that followed my previous surgeries and what I normally endured through the healing process always made it difficult for me to eat solid foods, and soup remained the staple of my meal plan.

But not today. Today was different.

Today I felt strong and replenished, and I wanted to try to eat something more solid.

We stopped at a restaurant, and as I ordered the whole left side of the menu, I salivated. I was soooo hungry for *real* food. When the server delivered my dinner, I wanted to feast, but I chose to carefully take my first bite and build up to whatever level my body allowed.

After a successful first bite, it was *Game On!*

My companion and I were shocked as I continued to eat everything in sight without pain or discomfort.

"Okay, I have no idea what this grounding phenomenon is, but I know that it's something special." In all my years of recovery from these repeated surgeries, I had never been able to comfortably swallow solids until after week four.

Once home, I immediately unpacked my new gifts and learned all about the products. That same night, I put the grounding mat on my bed and connected it, along with the pillowcases.

I was ready!

My parents stopped by to see how it went. I excitedly monopolized the conversation.

My dad interrupted.

"You're speaking?!"

What a huge moment for us, as I spoke in full tone with them; yet, when I left them in the morning, I was unable to speak. They were taken aback and left speechless.

With this new to me phenomenon, everything was about to change.

That evening, exhausted after all the events of the day, I slapped some patches on my hand and slept on my grounded bed. I looked forward to finding out what a whole night of grounding would do for me, and my stroke created insomnia.

Insomnia has become a massive part of my life. It's widespread for stroke survivors and those with brain injuries to experience this symptom long-term. I found insomnia to be one of the most annoying things I endured due to my stroke. I tried anything and everything to fix this issue, but nothing I found would do the trick.

Repeatedly, I woke up all hours of the night, lucky if I slept three hours in a row, and when I woke, I never felt rested. Every neurologist told me, "Learn to deal with sleeplessness." The only other option included heavy prescription medicine that made me feel like a zombie throughout the day and delayed my reaction time—out of the question for me.

Let me tell you, I have experienced some pretty unforgettable moments in my life... but this moment with grounding goes down in my personal history book. I went to bed just as I do every night. The only difference was that I was grounded. I woke up to the sun shining on my face and hearing the birds chirping.

Wait, wait, wait, what? It's morning!!!

I started chanting, *"It's daytime! It's daytime!"*

I woke up rested for the first time in years. My gratitude for this life change continued day after day. Now, completely sold on the Earthing healing phenomenon, I was obsessed!

From that day forward, I have been a huge advocate for grounding. I walk outside barefoot every day, every chance I get. It's funny, even though my neighbors always laugh at me, "there goes Brisa with no shoes on again," I always encourage them to try it. If they only knew the grand change this would create in their own lives!

My barefoot morning walks outside on the grass immediately calm down any anxiety in my body and regulate my nervous system. I also notice that when I'm grounded, I feel more connected with the earth and can take much deeper breaths. Overall, I just breathe better in general.

SINCE I BEGAN GROUNDING REGULARLY, in a year and a half, I have only had throat surgery once, as opposed to every 6-9 months. I honestly feel that I am continuously getting better and better every moment I am grounded. I have high hopes that one day, these surgeries will be a story from my past.

I recommend this simple modality to everyone! I genuinely believe in Earthing because of the profound effect on my recovery. No placebo effect there for me, just pure benefit.

Thank you, Clint Ober.[1]

1. Research References

9. Classification of EEG Signal for Body Earthing Application 2018
https://earthinginstitute.net/wp-content/uploads/2021/10/RahmanAl.EEG_for_Body-Earthing_Application-2018-1.pdf

14. One-Hour Contact with the Earth's Surface (Grounding) Improves Inflammation and Blood Flow—A Randomized, Double-Blind, Pilot Study 2015
www.scirp.org/Journal/PaperInformation.aspx?PaperID=58836
15The Effect of Grounding the Human Body on Mood 2015
prx.sagepub.com/content/116/2/534.full.pdf+html

18. Grounding the Human Body Improves Facial Blood Flow Regulation 2014
http://www.scirp.org/journal/PaperInformation.aspx?PaperID=51326#.VHDemfnF8SA

22. Emotional Stress, Heart Rate Variability, Grounding, and Improved Autonomic Tone: Clinical Applications 2011
https://earthinginstitute.net/wp-content/uploads/2016/07/Emotional-stress-study.pdf

30. The Biologic Effects of Grounding the Human Body During Sleep as Measured by Cortisol Levels and Subjective Reporting of Sleep, Pain, and Stress 2004
https://earthinginstitute.net/wp-content/uploads/2016/07/Cortisol-Study.pdf

42. Earthing: health implications of reconnecting the human body to the Earth's surface electrons.
https://pubmed.ncbi.nlm.nih.gov/22291721/

44. Electric Nutrition: The Surprising Health and Healing Benefits of Biological Grounding (Earthing).
https://pubmed.ncbi.nlm.nih.gov/28987038/

46. The effect of grounding the human body on mood.
https://pubmed.ncbi.nlm.nih.gov/25748085/

52. The biologic effects of grounding the human body during sleep as measured by cortisol levels and subjective reporting of sleep, pain, and stress.
https://pubmed.ncbi.nlm.nih.gov/15650465/

4

A SECOND CHANCE

CIRCULATION AND INFECTION

LINDA CERA

I've always considered myself a very spiritual person. As such, I lived a grounded life.

For me, being spiritually grounded is the foundation upon which everything in life is built. It's the most basic of basics: I experience life in touch with my body, surroundings, and, most importantly, myself. When grounded, I live in the present moment.

Grounding helps center me and hold me calm amidst life's stressors. Everything that moves around me feels peaceful and manageable.

Then in 2016, I heard about a different kind of grounding —Earthing.

I never really understood physical grounding until I experienced it firsthand; it changed my life.

I KNOW that if I had just read about the many benefits of Earthing, the impact wouldn't be the same—I needed to try it to appreciate it!

My hands-on moment came about in mid-December at a Chopra event in Carlsbad. A company contributed several zero-gravity, grounded recliners for people to test, which they did during the breaks.

As I worked at the convention, I overheard all the "oohs" and "aahs" about how everyone relaxed and fell asleep in those chairs.

I thought I'd check it out.

I plopped myself down in a chair, thought about the grounding I knew, and waited for the peace and tranquility to lull me to sleep.

The peace and tranquility I knew didn't come. My experience wasn't relaxing at all!

An intense tingling filled my body.

My heart raced.

My sitting in this chair grew more and more irritating every second.

When my left foot reached the level of throbbing, it hurt so much that I had to stop the process and get out of the chair.

What's happening to me? I questioned.

I mentioned my misfortune and pain to Clint, the company representative.

He considered my reaction and then encouraged me that perhaps if I continued grounding, it might boost my circulation and reduce my inflammation, which would help relieve my pain. And since I kept my shoes on, Clint had no idea of my foot's condition, nor just how right he was!

What started several months before as an irritation between two toes from wearing flip-flops developed into an allergic reaction. My toes reacted negatively to the antibacterial Band-Aids I used to comfort my irritated skin.

I visited a couple of dermatologists only to find that their prescriptions worsened my condition! The initial skin irritation morphed into a complete disaster.

My foot swelled, cracked, and oozed!

What Clint said made sense to me, so I purchased an Earthing mat, which I put on my sofa.

Within a week, I saw a difference—my skin started to heal from the improved circulation. My pain subsided, and I felt a sense of well-being that I can only describe as peaceful and calm.

It was amazing!

For the rest of the week, I sat on my mat every chance I got.

Not only did my foot feel better, but my entire body achieved a greater sense of relaxation. And even though it was December, which traditionally brought me a level of high stress, I felt incredibly calm and relaxed.

What a concept—I let my body heal itself by increasing my circulation.

This first powerful experience opened the door for Earthing to become a permanent part of my life. The Universal Mat in my home office gets used every day. I also travel with Earthing products to ground myself wherever I end up.

If you're new to the concept, I highly recommend you try it. Whether working at my desk, taking a break to walk outside, or even just sitting in my car, I make sure to take a few minutes to connect with the earth. It's an essential part of my self-care routine, so much so that I can't imagine not doing it!

What a difference a small change can make in your life. *You will never know how much change is possible until you experience it yourself!*[1]

---

1. Research References
    9. Classification of EEG Signal for Body Earthing Application 2018
    https://earthinginstitute.net/wp-content/uploads/2021/10/RahmanAl.EEG_ for_Body-Earthing_Application-2018-1.pdf
    14. One-Hour Contact with the Earth's Surface (Grounding) Improves Inflammation and Blood Flow—A Randomized, Double-Blind, Pilot Study 2015
    www.scirp.org/Journal/PaperInformation.aspx?PaperID=58836
    15The Effect of Grounding the Human Body on Mood 2015
    prx.sagepub.com/content/116/2/534.full.pdf+html
    22. Emotional Stress, Heart Rate Variability, Grounding, and Improved Autonomic Tone: Clinical Applications 2011
    https://earthinginstitute.net/wp-content/uploads/2016/07/Emotional-stress-study.pdf
    30. The Biologic Effects of Grounding the Human Body During Sleep as

Measured by Cortisol Levels and Subjective Reporting of Sleep, Pain, and Stress 2004

https://earthinginstitute.net/wp-content/uploads/2016/07/Cortisol-Study.pdf

42. Earthing: health implications of reconnecting the human body to the Earth's surface electrons.

https://pubmed.ncbi.nlm.nih.gov/22291721/

46. The effect of grounding the human body on mood.

https://pubmed.ncbi.nlm.nih.gov/25748085/

52. The biologic effects of grounding the human body during sleep as measured by cortisol levels and subjective reporting of sleep, pain, and stress.

https://pubmed.ncbi.nlm.nih.gov/15650465/

5

SURFACE TENSION

SHOULDER PAIN, STRESS, & ANXIETY

JENNIFER JOHNSON

The Inner Connection to Separation

Having grown up in Long Beach, California, one of those concrete jungles, I initially remained clueless about the benefits nature brings to life.

Then, as a teenager, the opportunity came to go horseback riding. I found a favorite trail that took me out by a little creek. There, in this little patch of beauty, I discovered my love for nature and an appreciation for its healing power.

Even before I knew what grounding was, I knew there was a connection between being near trees and feeling better. My love for the time I spent around trees and forests inspired me to make a special effort to go to the redwoods and stand on the ground under those silent giants. In that space, the soft earth and trees offered a unique sense of nurturing, and I connected effortlessly to the sacred space inside myself.

If you live in an urban area, like me, you're likely used to a concrete jungle where the cities have tall buildings that block natural light and views. When you live on the upper floors of these concrete giants, you develop isolation from your surroundings. Even with floor-to-ceiling windows or skylights, you still miss out on the natural light and beautiful views of a more rural area.

I happened to have a conversation with a woman from New York City. I recall her telling me that the sunlight in her apartment only came from reflections off the buildings next door. She explained that she could see this warm glow as the sun shone on every wall through the reflected light of the other structures around hers.

She brought a fascinating perspective to me and helped me see again how much appreciation I have for these little gifts in life. Unlike many others, this woman did not take something as familiar as the sun for granted.

This city dweller's perspective differed sharply from mine. Now, living in a small town without skyscrapers to block my view, I'm used to seeing the sky and the trees from my window. Seeing her experience as she lived in her urban environment amazed me. She appreciated the beauty of nature and told me that she liked to touch the leaves and foliage when she went outside. She found it calming to be in contact with them and dreaded being disconnected from nature. Because of my deep love and respect for trees, I related to her experience.

I know it's not always easy to see how everything is interconnected. But, if you can take a step back and look at the big picture, you may be able to find some solutions that can help improve your health. Methods like meditation, movement, and massage all have a way of reconnecting us to our inner selves, reducing the separation between us, nature, the earth, and healing. When you can't visit the trees, you can find a way to bring nature's peace to you.

This brings me to my first experience with grounding as a tool.

Surprisingly, I felt the power of being connected and grounded while seventeen stories up in a Las Vegas hotel. The method for this grounding experience appeared to me during a convention when I took advantage of a unique free giveaway—a grounding pillowcase.

That night in my room, unsure what to expect, I put the case on my pillow and went to sleep.

I woke up in the middle of the night vibrating. This grounded case created an extreme difference in my body. The intensity of the vibration kept me awake and forced me to set aside the pillowcase if I was going to have any chance of returning to sleep.

More than just discomfort, I held an awareness of the shift this grounding created.

Due to my sensitivity and my attunement to nature, the initial explosion of connection that flowed through my system drove me to distraction.

I needed to take it slow and spread the connection out over time to build up to the intensity of the benefit this grounded pillowcase allowed. Small increments supported this plan and allowed me to get used to the feeling of this unexpected change.

The Proof is in the Footing

As the Director of Mind and Body Programs at Chopra Global, a company that teaches people about the benefits of healthy living, my work spanned many fields, including massage therapy and meditation. My position allows me to express my passion for the benefits of a healthy lifestyle. I choose to help others find the same happiness and peace that is my daily gift to myself.

With that in mind, imagine my reaction when the opportunity arose for me to play a first-person role in a grounding study. There was no chance I would pass that up, especially when the testing was conducted by the one and only Clint Ober and his team.

The Chopra Center hosted the team for six weeks, where we witnessed the change Earthing brought to individual lives. This study was like no other previously conducted. Even though many studies gathered data on how grounding helped people heal, no one had yet looked into the benefits and support brought to the workplace and how these changes extended to therapists while they worked.

Clint set the stage for the project and brought thick Earthing mats that covered every inch of floor space in the massage rooms. When the practitioner came in to do their work, they stood with their shoes off.

Clients also moved through the space with their shoes off.

Every set of feet in the building encountered these mats, and this barefoot connection allowed everyone to reap the benefits continuously.

One goal of the team's work was to see the impact the Earthing mats could have on the workers' daily pain.

Surprisingly, massage therapists, who dedicate themselves to eliminating the pain in others, suffer chronic shoulder pain. The constant pressure, the push of energy into the recipient's body, and the push back into the therapist's arm from cellular resistance take a physical toll on their bodies.

For me, I paid attention to a second aspect, the impact on the practitioners' ability to hold sacred space. This aspect of massage therapy and energy work—their ability to remain grounded in the energies of the earth while they hold space for transformation and change—is essential. As they hold themselves centered and balanced, the process allows the clients to explore their emotions and heal their wounds.

During the very successful six weeks, information was gathered regarding the reduction in pain in the workers' bodies, measurable improvement in their focus and productivity, and increased ability to stay grounded with less effort while, at the same time, they helped the client to heal.

One of the participants in the study remained skeptical of grounding. She didn't believe that the mats brought any benefits. Despite this, she continued to work barefoot for the duration of the study.

At the end, when the mats were removed from the office, she noticed an increase in pain in her shoulder. Because of the gradual reduction and elimination of her pain, she had forgotten that the daily shoulder pain existed. Now, she's a firm believer.

.   .   .

FOR MYSELF, my transformation both encouraged and astounded me. Before the study, the idea that this connection may negatively affect my intuitive insights terrified me because of my sensitivities and spiritual awareness.

I rely on my intuition and ability to collect important information needed for myself and others to heal. I grew concerned that Earthing could keep me from receiving that information. Instead of reducing my intuition, I found that the support turns down the noise, removing the usual interference and static. Grounding makes it easier for me to bring in pertinent information.

CLIENTS AND FAMILY

Grounding helped me let go of stress and anxiety, reduce pain in my body and shoulders, heal from trauma, and find a sense of peace and calm in my life. In addition to these reliefs, I've also experienced an increase in energy and vitality, as well as an improvement in my quality of sleep. Moreover, my skin and hair have both looked better than ever, and I generally feel better overall.

I believe in grounding so much that I brought his transformative support to my clients and family.

When I work with people, I always use a grounding mat. This helps to improve the results we achieve together. Everyone assumes that the benefits they experience are from their massage and other treatments, but I believe that Earthing products play a huge role in their success.

I've seen similar changes to those I experienced myself with many of my clients. Grounding helps them let go of chronic pain, overcome anxiety and depression, and find more joy and happiness in their lives. Often, they report feeling more energetic and well-rested, in addition to a bounty of other benefits after starting their Earthing practice.

Even though the proof is there, one's family can be the last to turn around and join in on what we know works.

My husband, a professional weightlifter, endures intense strain on his body. When he was recovering from a herniated disc, he didn't want to believe me about the benefits of grounding.

Just to humor me, he tried one of my tools and wore the grounding belt to bed.

The following morning, he sat on the bed and said, "Wow, this surprisingly worked." Over time, his pain decreased because he discharged the energy that kept his muscles tense.

My mother-in-law is another perfect example of how Earthing products make all the difference. Her physical therapy routine demanded consistent effort, which always seemed to help for a little while. Yet, the benefits repeatedly wore off as her inflammation increased with movement. She stopped going to her appointments each time because of the pain it caused her.

Grounding easily and naturally reduces inflammation and thus reduces pain. As a passive exercise, using an Earthing tool gains some of the same long-term benefits of physical therapy without all the complex, painful effort.

For this reason, I find that it is much easier to have folks commit to trying a mat for a month instead of physically moving these painful body parts.

My mother-in-law is no exception. This woman, who is 72 years old, found relief from sitting in a grounded chair after just a few minutes. Her movement increased and the pain she had experienced for years reduced.

To my surprise, one day, I walked into the living room and found her sitting in the chair with her legs crossed, smiling from ear to ear.

"Wow - look at you!" I thought. She hadn't had the freedom to move her body like that in forever.

Sitting grounded reduced a lifetime of chronic inflammation. The chair became a revelation for her as years of pain and discomfort melted away. The experience solidified her belief in the power of grounding and its ability to help improve people's health.

REDUCE Overwhelm

A woman I treated for overwhelm found grounding an effortless way to return to a state of calm and center. I trained her on the benefits of using natural methods and Earthing tools. When she feels the beginning forces of her overwhelm or the pressure of her stressors, she goes to the mat to reground and breathe. Her daughter, who is autistic, also uses this technique to calm down when she starts to become overwhelmed. This technique works well for them as they center themselves and regain control.

We can get lost in what we're doing and end up in repetitive patterns that push us, stress us, and make us feel overwhelmed. Different methods of grounding break us out of our routine.

For the therapists that work with me, I often recommend a walk on the beach when they have a rough day. Spending time near water can be incredibly grounding and relaxing, especially if you're having a tough day. If you cannot get to the beach, try spending time near a river, lake, or fountain. The sound of moving water can be incredibly soothing and calming.

Self-massage is another helpful method for learning to connect to your body through touch. Breast massage reduces inflammation and improves lymphatic flow. When you develop a better body connection through self-massage, you gain a more vital, grounded connection, which allows for healing on a deeper level. This, in turn, can help improve the range of motion and quality of life while reducing stressors and the feeling of overwhelm.

Remember the trees. All of nature and the great outdoors bring a special connection to grounding.

If you can't get outside, you still need to pay attention to how you feel. Many people are disconnected from their bodies and what they experience in the world.

Many people struggle with chronic illness or chronic inflammation but don't realize that all their life's stresses contribute to these problems. They don't realize that their chronic pain can take them to dark places, making clear thinking difficult.

No one is there to tell them, "Hey, maybe you need to try this, implement this."

Because it's not always easy to see how everything is interconnected, take that step back and look at the big picture. *You can find solutions that can help improve your health and your ground with the earth.*[1]

————————————————————————

1. Research References

   8. Effects of Grounding (Earthing) on Massage Therapists 2018
   http://www.scirp.org/Journal/PaperInformation.aspx?PaperID=82706
   9. Classification of EEG Signal for Body Earthing Application 2018
   https://earthinginstitute.net/wp-content/uploads/2021/10/RahmanAl.EEG_for_Body-Earthing_Application-2018-1.pdf
   14. One-Hour Contact with the Earth's Surface (Grounding) Improves Inflammation and Blood Flow—A Randomized, Double-Blind, Pilot Study 2015
   www.scirp.org/Journal/PaperInformation.aspx?PaperID=58836
   15The Effect of Grounding the Human Body on Mood 2015
   prx.sagepub.com/content/116/2/534.full.pdf+html
   22. Emotional Stress, Heart Rate Variability, Grounding, and Improved Autonomic Tone: Clinical Applications 2011
   https://earthinginstitute.net/wp-content/uploads/2016/07/Emotional-stress-study.pdf
   30. The Biologic Effects of Grounding the Human Body During Sleep as Measured by Cortisol Levels and Subjective Reporting of Sleep, Pain, and Stress 2004
   https://earthinginstitute.net/wp-content/uploads/2016/07/Cortisol-Study.pdf
   42. Earthing: health implications of reconnecting the human body to the Earth's surface electrons.
   https://pubmed.ncbi.nlm.nih.gov/22291721/
   46. The effect of grounding the human body on mood.
   https://pubmed.ncbi.nlm.nih.gov/25748085/
   52. The biologic effects of grounding the human body during sleep as measured by cortisol levels and subjective reporting of sleep, pain, and stress.
   https://pubmed.ncbi.nlm.nih.gov/15650465/

MY DAY OF INFAMY

STAGE 4 ENDOMETRIOSIS & INFERTILITY

TAYA CRAYK-BONDE

November 3rd, 2016, is my day of infamy. Just 23 years old, this day forever changed my life.

On the drive home, I was freezing. So, I cranked up the heater even though the temperature outside was already warm. I figured I must be coming down with a cold or the flu—nothing serious to worry about. I felt worn out, so much so that all I could think about was getting to my bed, curling up, and going to sleep.

Finally, I snuggled up in bed with two heating pads and drifted off.

I woke up the first time Mom came in to check on me. An entire day had passed since I'd laid down. I got up and immediately knew something was wrong.

I couldn't physically stand up straight. It was as if someone had sewn my insides to create this 90-degree angle in my body. The excruciating pain sent me crouching down each time I tried to stand up straight.

"Mom, something is very wrong... I need to go to the hospital."

Mom knows I'm not one to ask to go to the hospital for pretty much anything, so she quickly took my temperature to get a baseline reading.

104.1

My mother didn't say another word. She hurriedly grabbed her shoes and keys.

In pain and folded over, I couldn't walk.

Everything continued in a dream-like state, blurry, moving slowly, like how I often feel that split second before falling asleep.

The hospital staff came to get me from my car. Thank goodness because every single step, every jarring movement, brought tears to my eyes.

Everything hurt.

The staff rushed me to an exam room, and in a few seconds, the tests began. With my symptoms, they worried about one thing—an ectopic pregnancy.

I told them they had to keep testing because I wasn't sexually active; it couldn't be an ectopic pregnancy.

They ran test after test after test.

An MRI with contrast showed a cantaloupe-sized mass in my abdomen. They found the mass attached to my uterus, left fallopian tube, left ovary, bladder, and a large portion of my intestines.

Following a quick conclusion that this could be cancerous, they rushed me to a trauma hospital two hours away. A surgeon and a gynecologist specializing in oncology awaited my arrival, ready to perform emergency surgery.

As one does before going under the knife, I signed away my life as I acknowledged all the possible risks. The risk that stood out above all the others was that I'd likely lose my bladder along with my reproductive organs on my left side.

Reading that, that was the moment it all became frightening.

As they wheeled me away from my parents, I choked back my tears of fear; I might never see them again.

I woke from the anesthesia and sobbed and shook uncontrollably. The physical pain was still excruciating, I felt out of control emotionally, and the effects of the medications compounded my distress.

No one filled me in on the outcome.

I didn't know how it went or what they saw or found.

And amongst all this angst, I wanted Mom and Dad next to me.

The staff sedated me to help with the pain.

Still alone and without my parents, I got some news from the gynecologist during one of my more lucid moments.

Because of the size of the mass, they opened me hip to hip. My scar would resemble a C-section incision, only longer. The fever, lethargy, and delirium I experienced occurred because of septic shock. Fortunately, they saved my bladder and left my damaged ovary and fallopian tube in place, hoping they might still function.

The doctor paused before telling me more.

The pause meant bad news was coming, and I held my breath.

"We sent the tissue to pathology," another pause, "Having never seen a mass quite like this one, I can't say for sure if it's cancerous or not."

He quietly left after letting me know the general surgeon needed to speak to me privately regarding the other findings.

The delay further shook me.

It took nearly a day for the general surgeon to come to my room. Thankfully, my mom waited with me to hear the update.

The surgeon arrived expressing only a minimal amount of the much-needed bedside manner for which I yearned.

"You have stage 4 endometriosis; I would even consider it to be worse than that. The worst case I have personally seen in my many years of opening people up. If you don't know what endometriosis looks like, picture dumping a large bowl of Elmer's Glue all over your insides."

His abrupt sharing put me off, and if that wasn't enough bad news, he added like it was nothing, "I'll send you to a fertility specialist," revealing that my overall fertility was at risk. "Yes, with the extent of your disease, I don't think it's going to be possible for you to conceive or even carry a child naturally. I would give it a 0-1% chance."

He spewed just one terrible thing out of his mouth after another. The details he shared about this disease's excruciating pain didn't phase me because I had already lived unknowingly with it for years. But his blunt delivery of how much destruction inflammation brings and the other horrible side effects tipped me over the edge.

"So, you will also need to see a pain therapist and, at the very least, be put on anti-inflammatories to help you tolerate the pain."

He hit me with a ton of bricks, then another ton, and another!

In a matter of a few days, everything in my life changed dramatically. My life went from being just a cancer scare to my owning this horrible, harrowing disease, AND I'm now being told I am infertile.

The *why me's* started piling up. *Why me, why this?*

Ever since I was a little girl, all I ever wanted was to one day be a mom, and to have a child that loved me as much as I loved my mom. To have that one-of-a-kind bond fulfilled my dream, my perfect experience that gave my life value.

With his careless words, all those dreams were stolen away.

The overwhelm that I felt sent me into a depression. As a young woman... being told that your body won't work how it's designed to can really affect your mental health.

It affected mine in the worst way.

A few weeks later, the pathology results finally returned benign. The most absolutely fantastic news to receive amid all the upheaval.

WHAT CAME NEXT WAS A NIGHTMARE. I didn't know yet that the battle had just begun. I didn't know that the surgery that saved me awakened a new monster.

PAIN. **Pain. Pain.**

Sharp, radiating pain every single day.

I was convinced the all-day-every-day pain must be the result of them accidentally leaving some surgical instrument inside me. I could not fathom anything else being the cause of such debilitating pain.

I hurt when I walked, when I moved, and when I shifted to get more comfortable, I hurt.

I spent agonizing days in bed, unable to get up.

After the surgery, my disease stepped into overdrive, and it worked overtime to replace the invasive tissue and mass that the doctors surgically removed. That doctor who told me I would need to see a pain therapist, I now realized, was trying to do me a favor. Even though I was against taking a bunch of pills, I did go on an anti-inflammatory regimen to try and dampen the sharpness of my daily pain. I figured I could tolerate most of it if I could get rid of the edge.

Let me try to help you understand endometriosis. Honestly, I don't think most doctors know much about endometriosis. Many don't have the knowledge they need to assist in the diagnosis. They also can't "officially" diagnose a patient until they open the patient up with surgery. Endometriosis is where the endometrium, the tissue that lines the inside of the uterus, grows outside of the uterus; surgery is the only way to see this occurrence.

In the years that preceded my surgery, I can't tell you how I struggled with pain related to my lower abdominal area, how often I saw a doctor who told me I imagined it, how many times they told me I just had irregular menstruation and irregular menstrual side effects.

Before my operation, not one doctor mentioned that these side effects were happening because of endometriosis or even that it was a possibility.

Typically, endometriosis affects the reproductive organs and the intestines, but it has been seen as far away as the lungs and brain. The cause of endometriosis is still unknown, and no one really knows why it happens, but with four stages—Minimal, Mild, Moderate, and Severe—many women struggle with this disease and don't even know they have it.

With all the pain I endured in the coming months, it didn't

surprise me that scans revealed that new growths took up the space of the excised one. Plans for future surgeries were made.

I saw doctor after doctor after doctor, seeking their best professional advice. Every time one gave me their opinion, I scheduled another appointment for a second opinion, and so forth. I saw fertility specialists, family practitioners, endocrinologists; you name it...not one, not two...I finally lost count after around sixteen doctors.

Each specialist echoed the last. They each told me that this painful disease, one with no pinpoint of cause or origin, had no actual treatment other than surgery after surgery to try and excise any growth or tissue, which most of the time leads to more aggressive growths and adhesions, guaranteeing the throes of the disease became more and more painful.

They always ended their instructions the same way: "You have to keep an eye on the disease for the rest of your life."

To top off the permanence of my sentencing, they also threw in facts about my fertility, how my condition affected it, and that I had no chance of conceiving. Zero.

By now, you might feel you have to join me in my sad, depressed state.

I felt discouraged.

I felt alone.

I felt my body broken and my health gone.

My body's betrayal left me angry.

I lived with pain in every way imaginable.

THE ONE THING that pushed me to continue my quest for answers with all these different doctors was that not one of them truly understood the disease, not really. They couldn't tell me what caused it. They couldn't tell me if there would ever be a cure for it or what I could do to help it. They kept repeating that I would have to rely on pain management and therapy, that I would have to try and combat the inflammatory issues that come with the disease, and that the only temporary relief people got was time spent pregnant. But there would never be any relief for me because my condition was in the later stages, affecting my fertility.

The repeated handoff of, "IF it had been caught earlier, you could have tried to conceive, with a small chance of becoming a mother before your condition reached this point," although well-meaning, hit me in my heart, each time a terrible repeated blow to hear.

I remained inconsolable.

FAST FORWARD

A year later, in November of 2017, my struggle continued. I relied on a steady dose of naproxen 4x daily to help keep the inflammatory side effects at a less severe level. My most common experience came at night when the pain woke me from sleep: my only recourse was pacing. I paced the room until I was completely exhausted, so exhausted that I didn't care how badly I hurt because, after wearing myself out, I would finally be able to shut my eyes until morning.

Pacing.

Every.

Single.

Night.

DURING THIS TIME, I had become a bit reclusive. I stopped seeing friends, and I avoided going out on dates. I didn't want to talk about it, and I didn't want to have to explain to a possible future boyfriend about my infertility. Because for me, I wasn't enough as a partner if I couldn't have children with my future husband. I treated myself unkindly during this time...I beat myself up and took responsibility for something entirely out of my control.

Then out of the blue, on November 10, 2017, I got a message on Facebook from Slater, a friend from high school.

Recently, he endured a life-altering loss and reached out to me for help in creating a memorial tattoo design. So, I helped.

Time passed, and my talks with him became an everyday thing.

These talks brought a very much-needed comfort, a comfort I didn't even conceive of being possible with the current level of pain and sadness I carried.

Often, in our conversations, we skipped the struggles; honestly, we talked about everything but our pain, which helped both our emotional healing. Slowly, over time, what we were going through came out during those in-depth talks.

He asked to meet. He believed he had something that would help alleviate my everyday pain.

On December 12, 2017, we met and sat at a booth in Applebee's. He pulled out this box and this mat and those little sticky pads. I had no idea what this stuff was, and my side-eye-squirrelly-look probably let him know that I thought there was no way this could be the answer to my prayers. So desperate for relief at that point, I figured, *Why not give it a try?*

He explained it thoroughly.

He explained Earthing and grounding and how connecting to the earth floods your body with negative ions that eliminate inflammation.

He didn't want me to rely on medication.

He knew in the long run that external reliance harmed the body.

He wanted me to try something natural, something I could have access to just by going outside, putting my bare feet onto the grass, into the sand, and being connected to the earth.

As he shared, the details made sense, how we had lost that connection when humans isolated themselves from the earth.

We isolate our feet by wearing shoes, living in insulated homes, and cutting ourselves entirely off from this natural phenomenon that the body needs.

Slater explained that the mat and sticky pads were tools to help me ground in my home. The mat, made of conductive material, gets plugged into the grounding port of an outlet; the same instructions apply to the patches he gave me.

So, that night at home, I unpacked the mat and plugged it in with nothing to lose. I placed it underneath my fitted sheet near my feet and put the patches on my belly, where the new growths had popped up inside. I crawled into bed and fell asleep.

I woke up to the sun shining through my window. I blinked my eyes several times, completely confused about how long I had slept. For the first time in months, I slept through the entire night without getting up to pace the pain away.

THAT SAME SLEEP-FILLED night was repeated and repeated and repeated!

IN THE COMING WEEKS, I stopped reaching for my multiple daily doses of Naproxen. Eventually, I stopped refilling my prescription. In only a couple of weeks, my worry over the permanence of medicine in my life faded like a bad dream.

With grounding, I also ended my need for follow-up surgery. The new growth never reached a stage that required surgical intervention. After five years of grounding, I never need to pace myself to exhaustion to ignore the pain so I can sleep.

The impossible became possible. Here I was, in late stage 4, and I could give my body a break from all the inflammation. Grounding made it possible to allow my body to heal and get a foothold on the disease.

To be pain-free every day.

To be able to get a whole night of rest.

To be able to get out of bed and get things done.

To skip the constant notice of side effects.

I am to the point where I question if I still suffer from stage 4 anymore.

The biggest thing that stunned me and my entire family and doctors came in September 2019. I announced my pregnancy. To share that I was expecting a baby changed my whole outlook on life, and for the father to be the love of my life, Slater, made my miracle complete.

Slater and I accomplished something we were told had a 0% chance of happening. With all my body had been through and all the time I spent worrying and being sad about my body failing me, those thoughts flipped in a matter of a moment with a single test.

Not only did I naturally conceive, but I also carried her to term and gave birth to our beautiful, healthy, and happy baby girl.

My extraordinary little miracle...made possible through grounding. [1]

---

1. Research References
9. Classification of EEG Signal for Body Earthing Application 2018
https://earthinginstitute.net/wp-content/uploads/2021/10/RahmanAl.EEG_for_Body-Earthing_Application-2018-1.pdf
14. One-Hour Contact with the Earth's Surface (Grounding) Improves Inflammation and Blood Flow—A Randomized, Double-Blind, Pilot Study 2015
www.scirp.org/Journal/PaperInformation.aspx?PaperID=58836
15 The Effect of Grounding the Human Body on Mood 2015
prx.sagepub.com/content/116/2/534.full.pdf+html
22. Emotional Stress, Heart Rate Variability, Grounding, and Improved Autonomic Tone: Clinical Applications 2011
https://earthinginstitute.net/wp-content/uploads/2016/07/Emotional-stress-study.pdf
30. The Biologic Effects of Grounding the Human Body During Sleep as Measured by Cortisol Levels and Subjective Reporting of Sleep, Pain, and Stress 2004
https://earthinginstitute.net/wp-content/uploads/2016/07/Cortisol-Study.pdf
36. The Effects of Grounding (Earthing) on Inflammation, Immune Response, Wound Healing, and Prevention and Treatment of Chronic Inflammatory and Autoimmune Diseases 2015
https://www.dovepress.com/articles.php?article_id=21001
41. The effects of grounding (earthing) on inflammation, the immune response, wound healing, and prevention and treatment of chronic inflammatory and autoimmune diseases.
https://pubmed.ncbi.nlm.nih.gov/25848315/
42. Earthing: health implications of reconnecting the human body to the Earth's surface electrons.
https://pubmed.ncbi.nlm.nih.gov/22291721/
46. The effect of grounding the human body on mood.
https://pubmed.ncbi.nlm.nih.gov/25748085/
52. The biologic effects of grounding the human body during sleep as measured by cortisol levels and subjective reporting of sleep, pain, and stress.
https://pubmed.ncbi.nlm.nih.gov/15650465/

7

A PATH FOR SPIRITUAL AWAKENING

GROUNDED YOGA, CHILDBIRTH, BREATH WORK, & AWAKENING

ASHLIE FLOOD

*B*arefoot and Brave
Nature presents me with a way to connect with something larger than myself, to feel I am part of the world instead of apart from it. Being in nature feels good for my soul.

While still existing in my conventional western mindset, my desire for connection brought me to my yoga practice. Before 2012, when I chose my independence, I attended guided yoga in fitness gyms and studios.

The first thing I did when I began practicing on my own was take it outside.

I didn't consider any reason for this other than my general desire to be outdoors. Liberated, I found I could care for my body's physical exercise needs without requiring more than a mat and some space. I craved the freedom this change brought and, with some planning, I kept the experience as natural as possible. I even did away with my rubber barrier in exchange for a handwoven, cotton creation, something unheard of in sticky-mat-addicted western yoga culture.

While seeking more natural ways to live and thrive, I strove to remove myself from western medical intervention. Further support for my park practice came from a holistic physician. This physician shared in passing the physiological benefits achieved when a person connects directly on the grass. Already active with the barefoot lifestyle I developed to heal a running injury, the concept breezed through my awareness without much care. Regularly outside with nothing on my feet, I knew this benefit to be mine and put no other thought into it.

A YEAR OR SO LATER, indoor grounding introduced itself to me as a birthday gift—a set of sheets for my bed. How putting a cord into a wall grounded me the same as living barefoot outside made little sense. Still grateful for the gift, I read Clint Ober's Earthing book that came with the sheet set. He explained that the connection we are looking to achieve is electrical.

The concept sold me through and through.

Between the studies that showed various physiological benefits, I understood how grounding somehow filled a gap in our health needs that currently focused on the simple concepts of diet and exercise to achieve wellness.

After I put the sheets on my bed, I initially noticed no difference, probably, due to my lifestyle of daily barefoot grounding. As many others share instances of miraculous healing, my story is devoid of such an experience. However, I find it rather interesting that I conceived my first son the same month I put the sheets on my bed, supporting our plan to become pregnant.

My first child was already growing inside of me, and I wanted to deliver my baby naturally and free from medication. This produced motivation and an opportunity to develop my ability to manage pain and discomfort from the inside out with a focused yoga practice.

And So It Is

Before the concepts of 'mindfulness' and 'meditation' grew into the science-validated buzzwords of today, they were considered far-fetched and lived only in the realms of spirituality. Although I practiced and studied yoga, as a front-line healthcare worker, these concepts remained very far from my practical western world. Even to this day, I do not incorporate or teach practices until I have learned of some scientific validation.

So, to move mentally and physically with these *new to me* concepts, I purchased a 108-bead mala, which I used to tangibly develop a meditation practice. The simple approach of sliding the beads between my fingers on every exhale until I completed the circle carried me forward, and I successfully reached my meditation and mindfulness goal.

My son was born free of medication or medical intervention, even within a hospital setting. While still a challenge for many mothers today, this was nearly unheard of at the time.

The birthing process itself brought me a tremendous spiritual experience. When you combine my desire to connect with the reality-bending experience of new motherhood, this combination transforms me into a completely new person from the inside out.

Following these changes, the concepts of atheism, which I used for years to shape my reality, no longer satisfied my thoughts. The new understanding raised my awareness. I experienced an elevated and intimate connection, knowing there is much more to this existence than meets our five explored human senses.

MY PLANNED PREGNANCY allowed me to stay home with our son. I settled into motherhood, my yoga practice continued to deepen, and I kept grounding all the while.

Soon after my son's first birthday, something changed in me.

I grew stir-crazy as a full-time mother. The helper, the teacher, and the healer in me needed an outlet. From my years in high school as a lifeguard and peer tutor to my 11-year tenure in direct patient care for a medical laboratory, I lived in service to the community.

I knew the tremendous gift of being with my son, and the intensity of the stay-at-home role was a fleeting one, and I wanted an outward purpose to focus on while simultaneously raising him.

Even though I enjoyed my former career as a medical lab assistant, I didn't want to return to it. With my newfound holistic approach to life, I found myself on the outskirts of our western medical system. I needed to contribute to my community's healing and thriving in both a meaningful and unconventional way.

As I sat with these ideas, and in a very synchronistic and nearly simultaneous fashion, I received both my first job offer to instruct yoga at a gym and a work-from-home position with the same company that created and sold the grounding sheets.

I gladly accepted both opportunities, and to balance the scales, I enrolled in my formal yoga teacher training.

EXPERIENCE **Your Science**

My desire for validation of a holistic connection led me on a personal journey. I chose to do something I call experiential science. Experiential science is the practice of trying things out for yourself to see if they work, then making an evidence-based decision. I believe you cannot truly know something until you have experienced it first-hand; your experience is infinitely more valuable than secondhand information.

While my understanding of the experiential science of grounding unfolded, so did my yoga journey. Through my formal teacher's training, I spent six months deep diving into traditional yogic texts and practices in the lineages of Hatha, Vinyasa, Iyengar, Anusara, and Kundalini.

Knowledge and experience together drove me deeper into my intuition.

I felt wonderful.

I felt my life expand.

But sadly, my skeptical western mind still warred with the concepts and disputed their validity.

Despite several transformative experiences during meditation and training, these deeper insights were quickly brushed aside, which left me in my realm of consciousness. My yoga practice remained very physical.

Content with the rationalization that my physical focus suited my clientele—the athletic gym-going type—I kept my practice and classes at this social, superficial level, yet, at the time, it felt authentic.

With my athletic view, I led strength-focused vinyasa classes indoors and on grounded mats. The support of the mats meant little to the practice participants, as nobody seemed to understand what the mats were doing.

The experience wasn't enough.

Like me, most of my students could not consciously feel the grounding effect, certainly not within the confines of an hour focused on big, busy sun salutations!

It simply wasn't possible to squeeze in enough education or awareness while leading a movement class to entice them to seek a grounded lifestyle outside the studio's walls.

My mission grew to include educating others on the importance of a grounded lifestyle.

IN CONJUNCTION with the grounding job, this new mission drew me into a deep dive to learn everything I could about earth grounding and how it impacts the human body. My science-based thinking devoured studies that showed grounding produced:

- better sleep
- reduced inflammation and pain
- improved balance
- increased strength and coordination
- mood elevation and enhancement
- reduced delayed onset muscle soreness
- faster wound healing

With every published study, the list continued to grow. I even found a yoga practitioner-specific study devised to show improved blood viscosity when practicing while grounded.

Multiple grounding studies showed improved HRV and autonomic tone, pulse rate, and respiratory rate, all of which are markers for nervous system health and adaptability.

I began focusing my learning less on yoga asana and more on the sensing aspects of human physiology because, to me, this was mind-blowing. If something so subtle as touching the earth impacted our mood and body's ability to maintain homeostasis, I must consider that gave credibility to, well, ALL energy healing modalities.

This same year, Stephen Porges' published his now famed *Polyvagal Theory*, which helped me understand how deeply the state of my nervous system impacts my ability to operate in homeostasis physically. In addition, my body's subconscious autonomic sense of safety affects how I think, make decisions, and relate with others.

Combine the science facts with the Vedic knowledge I gained during this time, and a path formed that allowed my mind to surrender, and I embodied the meditative practices.

Come late 2017, by obtaining a balance of mental understanding of energy and how the entire system works together, earth grounding on a near constant basis, and frequent meditative practices, I created a magic potion that led me to experience a spontaneous kundalini awakening—an activity I dismissed as unreal until I experienced it for myself.

My kundalini rising left me with a fresh experience in my human body. Because of my ongoing holistic practices, my body experienced a space of safety, which allowed me to release subtle, unconscious traumas and physical misalignments, shifting to a level of homeostasis previously unachieved.

Many benefits followed this rise and the creation of a fresh experience.

The way my skin felt to touch became much more sensitive. The way my body moved through space was much softer and more fluid.

And for the first time, I consciously sensed whether I was grounded or not.

After several years of frequently physically grounding myself, studying, and teaching about it, I now felt it!

The mystery fully revealed itself for the first time during a phone call. As I chatted, I wandered through my home and experienced a very ungrounded situation. Intuitively, I touched one of the many mats I kept lying around.

The tension I didn't even know I held dissipated in a strong wave of tingles across my neck and shoulders. My breath drew an automated sigh, and my whole body softened into a calmer state.

To this day, this calming is the sensation I notice when I return to homeostasis as someone who is grounded.

Lead **Another to Ground**

In addition to grounding, I continued to learn and experiment with self-regulation practices, typically different types of breathwork and meditation, tapping, cold exposure, eye contact and smiles with friendly faces, play, movement, and balance work.

Something that stands out to me about grounding amid this mix of nervous system regulation techniques is that it's the only one I found where there is no DO-ing required. Yes, of course, you need to ensure your body is grounded, but that's all: no mindfulness, no attention work, no breath focus, and no pushing out of your comfort zone.

If you're grounded, you're grounded, and your system is receiving benefits.

I began to question how I could help people get and understand its importance, whether they felt it or not.

These questions that plagued my mind started to keep me up at night.

I awoke during the wee hours of the morning, jotted down ideas, and developed not just ways to promote the act of practicing yoga while grounded but a detailed program to help practitioners understand the importance this connection plays for our nervous system.

This program's development began to shift how my yoga asana practice looked and felt. As I continued my asana self-exploration, I spent some time dabbling in shamanic and sound healing. Through these journeys, I learned to trust my intuition better and let my imagination wander and play.

This trust liberated me!

My ongoing experiences with kundalini led me to explore tantra yoga and some Hinduism. In many ways, the world felt fresh, and I sensed my surroundings in increasingly subtle, unfamiliar ways.

At the moment they occurred, these changes were soft and natural. When outdoors on the trail, I tapped into the energy of my environment. Animals stopped skittering in fear as my bare feet approached. Instead, they nonchalantly meandered away.

Unleashed dogs began joyfully approaching me, knowing they had found a new friend.

I sensed an unspoken, unifying conversation with every living thing in my surroundings.

After learning about and believing in source consciousness, I arrived at a visceral understanding of the interconnected reality of existence.

With this tremendous shift, my yoga teaching also began to change.

Delighted, I bore witness to countless 'aha' moments as practitioners began to relate to themselves in more intimate ways. I witnessed as yogis reinforced and reinvigorated their practice.

To my delight, I've seen Grounded Yoga practitioners begin sharing grounding education on their social media pages!

In grounding, I discovered not only my healing and awakening but also achieved my life's work. My plan to help more people get grounded and tap into the state of their nervous system is working!

IF WE WANT to shift our society's collective toward a state of healing for both the planet and humanity, start by taking one barefoot step on the earth.[1]

1. Research References

9. Classification of EEG Signal for Body Earthing Application 2018
https://earthinginstitute.net/wp-content/uploads/2021/10/RahmanAl.EEG_for_Body-Earthing_Application-2018-1.pdf

14. One-Hour Contact with the Earth's Surface (Grounding) Improves Inflammation and Blood Flow—A Randomized, Double-Blind, Pilot Study 2015
www.scirp.org/Journal/PaperInformation.aspx?PaperID=58836
15The Effect of Grounding the Human Body on Mood 2015
prx.sagepub.com/content/116/2/534.full.pdf+html

16. Grounding the Human Body during Yoga Exercise with a Grounded Yoga Mat Reduces Blood Viscosity 2015
http://www.scirp.org/Journal/PaperInformation.aspx?PaperID=55445#.VSa19_nF_7A

22. Emotional Stress, Heart Rate Variability, Grounding, and Improved Autonomic Tone: Clinical Applications 2011
https://earthinginstitute.net/wp-content/uploads/2016/07/Emotional-stress-study.pdf

30. The Biologic Effects of Grounding the Human Body During Sleep as Measured by Cortisol Levels and Subjective Reporting of Sleep, Pain, and Stress 2004
https://earthinginstitute.net/wp-content/uploads/2016/07/Cortisol-Study.pdf

42. Earthing: health implications of reconnecting the human body to the Earth's surface electrons.
https://pubmed.ncbi.nlm.nih.gov/22291721/

46. The effect of grounding the human body on mood.
https://pubmed.ncbi.nlm.nih.gov/25748085/

52. The biologic effects of grounding the human body during sleep as measured by cortisol levels and subjective reporting of sleep, pain, and stress.
https://pubmed.ncbi.nlm.nih.gov/15650465/

8

EARTH HOLDS THE WAY TO HEAL

AUTOIMMUNE DISEASE, SENSITIVITY, & NERVE PAIN

CHRISTINE CONTINI

*T*he day my six-year-old daughter found me on the bathroom floor, unable to move eight feet to my bed without help, I knew I must increase my efforts to find an answer, a solution to the destruction Multiple Sclerosis brought to my body.

I took all the medication the doctors prescribed. I used daily self-injections. I forced movement of my failing body. I tried every piece of traditional advice I came across.

The limited relief I achieved from my constant pain, my attempts to reduce uncontrollable over-elevated stress reactions, and endless fatigue weren't enough. My family needed more from me, and I focused on the belief that I must get better.

I never played the poor me card. Instead, I did the impossible—I opened my mouth and talked to strangers. Communication was beyond uncomfortable, and still, I started a conversation with anyone, anywhere, any time someone made eye contact. We talked about what it meant to be well and how they or someone they knew achieved wellness. If the answer to wellness existed for my condition, I would find it.

I listened to them all.

I devoured huge quantities of information, and I believed every tidbit counted.

I tried unheard-of techniques that people secretly passed to me.

I read books by people who healed themselves from Multiple Sclerosis.

I studied science, metaphysics, and Buddhism; I researched each opportunity and put that opportunity into action. Every piece brought me closer to my goal of being well.

I admit that the constant effort to achieve wellness wore me down. Still, I kept at it.

During a particularly quick conversation, a lady at a doctor's office pulled a magazine out of her bag and told me to take it home. She said I would find what I was looking for in the pages. Excited that night, I got into bed and began to read. The articles seemed to have all the usual things, nothing new.

Disappointed, I set the folded periodical on my nightstand and slept.

When I woke up with my head hanging over the edge of the bed, I opened my eyes to find the magazine on the floor. Staring me in the face was an article about reducing stress. "Get a hobby," it said, "find an outlet," it encouraged, "get outdoors," it insisted.

I lay there with my face still hovering over the print and went through my routine of trying to bend my frozen limbs and fingers. Just as my vision turned black due to the unbearable pain, I caught sight of the one thing I thought I could do on the get outdoors list —gardening.

Memories of a seven-year-old me with plants in my room popped up. Gosh, I adored everything about those plants. I appreciated the hours spent collecting glass from the empty lot next door to earn the recycling money I needed to buy them. I loved that they were the first things I saw when I woke up. I cherished that I started my day off by talking to them from my bed and similarly ended my night.

The joy I felt for those memories took away some of the pain in my stomach.

While I waited several seconds for my vision to return, I stayed focused on gardening. I appreciated the idea that it would bring me joy and that I would find some relief by reducing stress.

In my current condition, gardening still seemed like a challenge but compared to hiking and swimming, and things that took me far from the safety of home, gardening remained the most doable. I figured I could sit on the ground and go as slowly as needed, and if I had everything within my reach, I could do that.

My kids helped me get everything set up and ready before they hopped on the bus for school.

With my brilliant mind destroyed due to the demyelination of my nerves and the many plaques that cut through my brain, every thought took more effort. *That's okay,* I comforted myself. *I have this magazine here to guide me.*

I sat down to begin. Even though the granules of dirt against my skin hurt as I sat on the ground in my shorts, I stayed there. Everything hurt my skin. Clothes hurt my skin. Hugs hurt my skin. Temperature changes hurt my skin. The pain distracted me as I read, so I read the first paragraph five or six times before I did what it instructed.

They told me to dig in the earth with my hands.

In my current state, the feeling of dirt on my hands, well, made me cry uncontrollably. I knew this fact; it wasn't going to be a new experience, and still, I pulled off my gloves. I dug into the soil in front of me and pulled the earth towards me until it covered my knees and the sides of my legs, where I could easily reach it.

I sat there in the dirt, tears streaming down my face while I sifted through the soil with my bare hands, preparing the earth so I could add my seeds. The directions said that proper soil preparation guaranteed the plants a safe and healthy place to grow. It took me about two hours to prepare an area of my garden of 3x1 feet. Then, exhausted, I moved to the lawn chair the kids had set out for me, and I fell asleep.

As the day passed, the shade of the pine tree no longer covered me, and I woke with the sun on my skin.

The sun, which generally hurts my skin, did not! The dirt on my hands seemed less painful than before.

The article guaranteed that connecting to the earth would change my body's stress level and a more relaxed body would feel less pain. I tried so many things that made promises and guarantees that were never delivered. I didn't expect this to work, and I felt blessed that because I tried everything, something finally did —grounding.

In addition to other alternatives to bring about wellness, I spent two or three hours every day in my garden for a year. Life changed, and after several years, I healed from Multiple Sclerosis. And as life often does, by 2008, I moved on from that pain, that struggle, and I forgot how Earth's masterful presence helped me find everything I needed to be well.

In 2018, things changed. I moved from wellness back to sickness. After enjoying the freedom of good health for several years, I returned to bed. Besides getting out of bed to eat or go to the bathroom, the only exercise I managed for four months was the short walk to my saltwater swimming pool. As I eased into the water each day, I felt an instant change in my health. Yet, after an hour of moving and exercising in my pool, I returned to exhaustion.

In addition to spending an hour every day in the grounding support of my pool, I meditated, worked on my mental and emotional baggage, and leaned into the wellness techniques I relied on from my past, things that worked when nothing else did.

Survival took constant effort.

My thoughts focused on the return of my pain and my inability to function, and their constant presence created an unbearable reality. I forced a shift to create change. As each thought reappeared, I dismissed the negative beliefs that pointed to a permanent relapse into Multiple Sclerosis. If I relaxed my mental control for even a minute, my heart raced, and my breath quickened. My body knew no comfort, only struggle.

I refocused on gratitude.

I changed the parts of life I held as stress into beautiful blessings.

Eventually, I started to feel better. Although not a cure, my efforts greatly improved my quality of life, level of joy, and ability to withstand the continued change in my body.

Still, survival took constant effort.

At the end of summer, I no longer ventured into our pool. By mid-October, the doctor had ordered me to be admitted to the hospital. They concluded that in addition to some blood and iron issues, the tests confirmed two more autoimmune diseases—Sjogren's and Rheumatoid Arthritis.

As the universe tends to open our path to destiny before us when we are ready, I ran into Elisabeth Hoekstra's book on BioHacking. In her book, she mentioned grounding. Her sharing of how the ocean grounds our bodies piqued my interest, and the comparison between my pool and the saltwater sea hit home.

Elisabeth used the ocean whenever she could during her travels and grounded herself in her new location. If she couldn't get to the water, she used grounding patches on her hands or feet to reground herself, eliminate jet lag, and reconnect to the earth.

Inspired, I opened the web page to make my purchase. I ordered a packaged set for me and another for my daughter, who constantly traveled and had symptoms that showed her need to ground.

The ground tester revealed every outlet in my RV as double red. So, my partner ran an extension cord from the construction power pole to the RV to properly connect the products to the ground.

The entire RV lacked ground!

That night, I slept sandwiched between the Earthing Mat and the pillowcase, which my family thought was strange initially, but my rapid improvement brought them around. They, too, began using the mats to help with their overall feeling of body stress and pain.

I pieced together more of this exciting puzzle as my brain fog cleared.

This return to gradual sickness came after moving. We moved from our home, where I spent a lot of time in the park or in our back-yard, to a piece of property we owned.

Instead of a house, we lived in an RV while we built on our land.

Instead of my regular barefoot grounding, I wore shoes all day because I lived on a construction site.

Because of the change in living space and lack of previous comforts, I just didn't meditate as often.

Extenuating circumstances took my year of RV living and dragged it out into three. By the second year, my hair had begun falling out, and a bald spot developed at the crown of my head. Another memory took me back to before I got sick with Multiple Sclerosis; in the beginning, I noticed my hair started falling out.

I believed hormones were the cause, so I questioned it very little. I wish someone would have made the correlation between my hair loss and the need for grounding for me and saved me a lot of time and suffering.

After about a month of living on my grounding mat, my hair stopped falling out.

LIKE MOST PEOPLE, for me, wellness requires a combination of mental, emotional, and physical support. I would not be well without grounding as a permanent piece of my puzzle.

Mother Earth, thank you for this precious gift of connection.[1]

---

1. Research References
      9. Classification of EEG Signal for Body Earthing Application 2018
      https://earthinginstitute.net/wp-content/uploads/2021/10/RahmanAl.EEG_
      for_Body-Earthing_Application-2018-1.pdf
         14. One-Hour Contact with the Earth's Surface (Grounding) Improves Inflam-
      mation and Blood Flow—A Randomized, Double-Blind, Pilot Study 2015
      www.scirp.org/Journal/PaperInformation.aspx?PaperID=58836
      15The Effect of Grounding the Human Body on Mood 2015
      prx.sagepub.com/content/116/2/534.full.pdf+html
         22. Emotional Stress, Heart Rate Variability, Grounding, and Improved Auto-
      nomic Tone: Clinical Applications 2011

https://earthinginstitute.net/wp-content/uploads/2016/07/Emotional-stress-study.pdf

30. The Biologic Effects of Grounding the Human Body During Sleep as Measured by Cortisol Levels and Subjective Reporting of Sleep, Pain, and Stress 2004

https://earthinginstitute.net/wp-content/uploads/2016/07/Cortisol-Study.pdf

36. The Effects of Grounding (Earthing) on Inflammation, Immune Response, Wound Healing, and Prevention and Treatment of Chronic Inflammatory and Autoimmune Diseases 2015

https://www.dovepress.com/articles.php?article_id=21001

41. The effects of grounding (earthing) on inflammation, the immune response, wound healing, and prevention and treatment of chronic inflammatory and autoimmune diseases.

https://pubmed.ncbi.nlm.nih.gov/25848315/42. Earthing: health implications of reconnecting the human body to the Earth's surface electrons.

https://pubmed.ncbi.nlm.nih.gov/22291721/

44. Electric Nutrition: The Surprising Health and Healing Benefits of Biological Grounding (Earthing).

https://pubmed.ncbi.nlm.nih.gov/28987038/

46. The effect of grounding the human body on mood.

https://pubmed.ncbi.nlm.nih.gov/25748085/

52. The biologic effects of grounding the human body during sleep as measured by cortisol levels and subjective reporting of sleep, pain, and stress.

https://pubmed.ncbi.nlm.nih.gov/15650465/

9

THE SHORT WALK TO WATER

ENERGY FLOW, STRESS REDUCTION, &
BODY ALIGNMENT

PATRICIA HACKER

*L*iving in Southern California, I often find myself at the beach. One of my favorite things is looking around at all the different people. Every day you see doctors, people in business suits, blue-collar workers, and your average beach-faring individual.

Everyone congregates to sit in the sand and dip their feet into the ocean. For some, their attraction to the beach is just the view. It's gorgeous and calming. For me, I question beyond the simple expression of beauty and consider why so many are drawn to spots of nature. Humans are connected to nature, even when we don't realize it.

It might surprise you that our divine power and purpose can become more apparent when we are connected to Earth. The natural flow of energy radiates through the ocean, which makes it a perfect spot to deepen your genuine connection.

My work on a wellbeing app, where I found new ideas, products, and ways to help Deepak spread the teachings of wellbeing, and self-care, brought me to my intersection with grounding as a tool. As the product manager of the Chopra Center, I met Clint and Olivia when they came in to share their Earthing line.

They shared how the connection to earth relieves stress, brings the physical form back into alignment, reduces inflammation, strengthens our ability to meditate, and more. Their products and their presence seemed like a natural fit. It was as if the Chopra Center found a piece of the puzzle when we met with Clint and Olivia.

The quick and noticeable change I experienced while using the Earthing support shocked me. When they placed one of the patches on my back, I immediately felt my energy begin to flow.

It was surreal.

It's hard to describe, but it felt "right."

That night I took home a grounding band, and I remember that my sleep that night allowed me to wake fully rested. I have been hooked ever since.

I implemented the Earthing products into my life to give my body the best chance possible at being the healthiest version of self in both physical form and mind. Because of this desire, I now keep a universal mat under my desk and use it daily.

I tell everyone I meet about all its benefits. I love how it easily and quickly made obvious changes in my life and the lives of many others.

One of my favorite stories to share includes an older woman in her late 70s and her daughter. I met them at the Chopra Event in Carlsbad. The mother was in a wheelchair and had been there for quite some time. We had her try the grounding chair, and as she sat there, we chatted a bit, and then they went on their way.

The next day, I was shocked to see the mother walking over to us with the assistance of a walker. Her daughter appeared very excited.

The daughter always kept a walker in her trunk, just in case her mother wanted to use it. This was the first time her mom requested she take it out for her to walk in over a year. Mom felt so good after her short session in the chair the day before that she wanted to try using her walker to get around.

On day three of the event, the woman again sat in the grounding chair and fell asleep. We let her rest. Suddenly, she stood up and walked unassisted to the restroom!

What a joy-filled story! I am eternally grateful for being a part of this practice, where I see firsthand the changes in lives.

Back at the Chopra Center, we often attracted people who struggled with relaxing while they learned meditation techniques. It was tough for them to calm themselves and create an environment that allowed them to get into the zone to meditate correctly.

Typically, in meditation or yoga, we help them through breathwork practices. Even then, many still struggle with the different techniques used to shut off their minds and just focus on their bodies.

We found that when we used grounding and Earthing products as part of our classes, people could relax more easily and get into the mindset to benefit from the instructions and practice.

The gift these products bring to our indoor lives continues to be incredible. Occasionally, I sit in one of the meditation chairs for an extra boost. Still, even with these life-changing products, my favorite method of grounding continues hands down to be walking along the beach.

Being in nature, with my feet in the water, the sand between my toes, and the natural elements of Mother Earth around me, is my oasis.[1]

---

1. Research References
    4. The Effects of Grounding on Meditation Quality: A Preliminary Study Report 2019 (abstract)
    https://earthinginstitute.net/the-effects-of-grounding-on-meditation-quality-a-preliminary-study-report/
    9. Classification of EEG Signal for Body Earthing Application 2018
    https://earthinginstitute.net/wp-content/uploads/2021/10/RahmanAl.EEG_for_Body-Earthing_Application-2018-1.pdf
    14. One-Hour Contact with the Earth's Surface (Grounding) Improves Inflammation and Blood Flow—A Randomized, Double-Blind, Pilot Study 2015
    www.scirp.org/Journal/PaperInformation.aspx?PaperID=58836
    15The Effect of Grounding the Human Body on Mood 2015
    prx.sagepub.com/content/116/2/534.full.pdf+html
    22. Emotional Stress, Heart Rate Variability, Grounding, and Improved Autonomic Tone: Clinical Applications 2011

https://earthinginstitute.net/wp-content/uploads/2016/07/Emotional-stress-study.pdf

30. The Biologic Effects of Grounding the Human Body During Sleep as Measured by Cortisol Levels and Subjective Reporting of Sleep, Pain, and Stress 2004

https://earthinginstitute.net/wp-content/uploads/2016/07/Cortisol-Study.pdf

42. Earthing: health implications of reconnecting the human body to the Earth's surface electrons.

https://pubmed.ncbi.nlm.nih.gov/22291721/

46. The effect of grounding the human body on mood.

https://pubmed.ncbi.nlm.nih.gov/25748085/

52. The biologic effects of grounding the human body during sleep as measured by cortisol levels and subjective reporting of sleep, pain, and stress.

https://pubmed.ncbi.nlm.nih.gov/15650465/

10

THE PROOF IS IN THE PAIN RELIEF

SORE THROAT & BROKEN LEG

SAMIA MCCULLY

My six-year-old woke with a sore throat, her tonsils so swollen they were almost touching. Her pain, audible in her voice, was reflected in her grumpy, tired expression.

Oh no! This was not good—a sick child on the Fourth of July when I expected 25 people over for a party? With only seven hours till the party kickoff, I wracked my brain—what could fix her throat in such a short amount of time and save me from canceling the party?

I decided to go to my office one more time. You see, I ordered a product that could change everything. Inspired by Olivia Ramirez Smith, whom I met at a conference, I felt pulled for a second time in my life to look at grounding as a resource. During the event, I sat down with Clint and Olivia at lunch and asked them a million questions. They were both so generous with their time and knowledge for almost an hour, and I left that lunch full of excitement. I immediately purchased Earthing mats and other grounding products for my patients and my family.

Not expecting anything since the box had yet to arrive the day before, all I could do was hope it came after I left the office.

Yes! The shipment arrived.

I placed an urgent call to Olivia and asked her how best to use the products for my daughter's throat.

"Put the patches on her neck as close to her tonsils as possible."

Each sticky patch consisted of a metal disc that needed to be in contact with the skin. I made sure the cords were plugged into my house's electrical ground and the other end was clipped onto the discs. I kept the cables untangled while she lay on a lounge chair outside. I tried to get her to keep her feet on the patio for even more grounded support. At only six, her attempt to hold this pose was unsuccessful. All the pressure was on the Earthing tools to perform.

For extra comfort, I used essential oils on her throat and allowed her to binge-watch Netflix for the next six hours.

By the time our guests started to arrive, her tonsils were less swollen, and she was energetic, with her throat pain reduced and her voice normal.

It worked! I was impressed, but I needed to see more to be convinced. It might all be a coincidence.

FORTUNATELY, the summer was ripe for grounding experiences.

Everyone in my house started sleeping on mats that very night.

My kids fell asleep quicker and slept deeper.

My husband stopped getting as hot at night, which helped him sleep better, too.

On the other hand, I still woke up multiple times a night, frustrated that these sleeping benefits somehow skipped over me. Where was my comfort, my peace of mind to wake up more rested? Why didn't these mats have the same effect on me?

Three weeks later, we went on vacation. I stripped the grounding mats off our beds and put them in my suitcase. We used them at the hotel, and I slept through the night for the first time in nine years since giving birth to my first child.

It felt great.

More importantly, the full night's sleep remained consistent.

Now, convinced that the mats were working, you might think this was enough, but it still wasn't.

Raise your hand if you are like me, always a skeptic. I needed to know why the tool didn't work for me right away when it worked for everyone else in my family. I needed more proof.

Little did I know, the proof I sought was about to hit me head-on. I asked for and received it.

ON MONDAY, my son, Max, went to the skatepark with some friends. I later got a call from the father; he feared Max had hurt himself during a fall.

Max was lying on the couch when I arrived with his leg propped up. I helped him to the car and brought him home.

For three days, I helped him to the bathroom and wherever else he needed to go. He rested with the grounding patches on his leg the whole time. Other than the inability to walk, he seemed fine.

On Wednesday, I decided that since my son wasn't walking, I would take him to urgent care the next day. With three kids, it was like a field trip to pile them into the car, drive off to Urgent Care, and then wait while they took Max away for an x-ray. The noisy waiting room was full of people. My young kids were antsy, and I grew impatient.

I told myself everything was okay, and with nothing wrong, we would go home and have lunch as soon as Max checked out fine.

When the X-ray technician finally called us back, I nearly fainted at the sight of the images.

Max snapped his tibia and fibula in half! Both long bones in his lower leg were broken, not even touching each other.

"Max may need surgery if they can't get the bones close enough." shared the doctor. As the blood drained from my head, I had to lie on the floor, my heart racing. I felt terrible for not bringing him earlier.

After a few minutes, I pulled myself together.

My neighbor came and picked up my two younger kids so I could focus solely on my wounded child.

My next stop, the pediatric emergency room at Stanford. I drove, still terrified and confused as to why Max hadn't been in pain all this time. He hadn't had any swelling over the last three days.

At Stanford, after 16 x-rays, 10 hours, and the casting complete, I waited for Max to come out of the sedation needed to move his bones into place.

"You're going to be in pain!" These were the words the supervising doctor gave the resident and me to repeatedly tell Max as he woke up.

But that didn't happen.

No pain.

And Max never needed the prescription painkillers.

And he never complained of any pain.

WHEN, after four weeks, the time came to reduce the cast, the new molding stopped just below the knee.

Max made plans for that same day, so right after the appointment, I dropped him off to attend a birthday party.

When I went to pick him up, his red, swollen knee caught my attention. A closer look showed what appeared to be an infection. While wearing the higher cast, Max scratched the back of his knee with a hanger; he must have scratched too deeply and left himself vulnerable to infection.

By the time we arrived home, the swelling had increased nearly twice as much, and his pain had approached an unbearable level.

My medical training caused me to panic. He might have had cellulitis, which required IV antibiotics.

Instead of joining me in my panic, my sweet boy, even in pain, kept a clear head. Tear-eyed, he encouraged me, "Mom, get the patches."

I plugged in the patches, put them on either side of his knee, and waited. His face changed from one of pain to surprise as he felt the pins and needles sensation, which meant the patches went to work on his knee.

"You're not going to believe this, but it doesn't hurt anymore," he shared.

Shocked, I couldn't believe the pain went away so quickly.

Grounding worked - there was no ambiguity. My son had spent much of the summer telling me to stop talking about grounding, and here was the proof it worked. Maybe I shouldn't have been so smug and satisfied, but GROUNDING WORKED!

And now, he, too, was convinced without a doubt.

We both were.

THESE FANTASTIC EXPERIENCES make me a huge advocate for grounding.

One habit I adopted after the conference with Clint and Olivia is going barefoot outside whenever possible. If I ever have a headache or I am run down, I'll go outside into my backyard in shorts and a tank top and lie down with as much exposed skin as I can or make sure I have on natural fibers. I always recover within about ten minutes.

Whenever I feel stressed or overwhelmed, I make sure to ground myself.

IN MY WORK life as a Naturopathic Doctor, we use grounding during patient treatment sessions. Each patient receives a Universal Mat and watches the Earthing documentary. Just like breathing clean air, drinking pure water, eating organic foods, and getting sun, I make it clear that grounding is an essential part of a healthy life.

According to my patients, the sheets help them remain more grounded and calm. Additionally, their pets will not let them sleep alone and will always want to be on the bed with them. They take this as a sign that the pets also benefit from the mats.

Even though not everyone can feel it, everyone benefits from Earthing products.

It's incredible how something as simple as connecting to the earth can positively impact our health and well-being.[1]

1. Research References

9. Classification of EEG Signal for Body Earthing Application 2018

https://earthinginstitute.net/wp-content/uploads/2021/10/RahmanAl.EEG_for_Body-Earthing_Application-2018-1.pdf

14. One-Hour Contact with the Earth's Surface (Grounding) Improves Inflammation and Blood Flow—A Randomized, Double-Blind, Pilot Study 2015

www.scirp.org/Journal/PaperInformation.aspx?PaperID=58836

15The Effect of Grounding the Human Body on Mood 2015

prx.sagepub.com/content/116/2/534.full.pdf+html

22. Emotional Stress, Heart Rate Variability, Grounding, and Improved Autonomic Tone: Clinical Applications 2011

https://earthinginstitute.net/wp-content/uploads/2016/07/Emotional-stress-study.pdf

30. The Biologic Effects of Grounding the Human Body During Sleep as Measured by Cortisol Levels and Subjective Reporting of Sleep, Pain, and Stress 2004

https://earthinginstitute.net/wp-content/uploads/2016/07/Cortisol-Study.pdf

42. Earthing: health implications of reconnecting the human body to the Earth's surface electrons.

https://pubmed.ncbi.nlm.nih.gov/22291721/

46. The effect of grounding the human body on mood.

https://pubmed.ncbi.nlm.nih.gov/25748085/

52. The biologic effects of grounding the human body during sleep as measured by cortisol levels and subjective reporting of sleep, pain, and stress.

https://pubmed.ncbi.nlm.nih.gov/15650465/

11

THE COLD DOESN'T BOTHER ME ANYMORE

ARTHRITIS PAIN, PLANTAR FASCIITIS, & MIGRAINES

DENISE MADRID

I am blessed.

I am blessed with five exceptional children.

I am blessed to live in one of nature's greatest masterpieces, the mountains!

And I am blessed to have found grounding. Grounding has changed everything for me.

I RAISED my children in the mountains. It has been my honor to share this masterpiece of nature with them, surrounded by such soul-enriching beauty each day. Living in the mountains is a dream come true, a natural paradise on Earth.

As a family, we spent time exploring nature and enjoying all our environment had to offer, from the beautiful sunset mountain views that led to star-filled night skies to the lush green trees that provided cover for all types of weather.

For me, the trees brought a special comfort. I remember long days when I worked hard outside on my land. On those warm summer days, the trees allowed through their branches the ample sunlight that I needed. I needed an extra soothing connection as I wrestled with pain from Plantar Fasciitis, sinus headaches, or difficulty breathing. Still, I loved my mountain lifestyle.

In the winter, it gets cold in the mountains.

The lower temperatures exacerbated my arthritis, which made walking through snow or lifting groceries from the car into our home nearly impossible. In the cold, my arthritis crippled me with painful flare-ups that made it difficult to get out of bed.

When the temperature reaches freezing, every bone in my body aches and normal function threatens to cease. However, I never gave up or let the pain control me. Because I am blessed, I continued to push through and fight. I knew that I'd be in an even worse state if I didn't.

On a medium day, the push through my pain kept me focused, but on a terrible day, that effort exhausted me.

Fortunately, after confiding in a friend about my years of struggle, she introduced me to the solution for pain relief—grounding. She explained how physical changes throughout different stages of our lives bring about pain, hormone imbalances, and inflammation. Earthing reduces the impact of these stressors.

With this introduction, my life permanently changed.

I started using mats, sheets, and pillowcases while I slept. Amazingly, these changes managed to reduce a myriad of ailments:

- It helped me breathe easier
- My headaches are gone!
- Cleared up sinus infections
- Improved my sleep, making it more restful

Before, when I slept, my face got all blocked up inside with these yucky air sacs that didn't want to go away on their own. With Earthing support, my sinuses stopped being blocked, my headaches disappeared, and my breathing eased up. Now, I sleep like a baby.

Additionally, my arthritis has become non-existent. I am free of pain and inflammation. Because my arthritis is managed, I no longer dread the cold of winter.

Grounding is wonderful. I swear by it.

Before a planned trip, I suffered from a Plantar Fasciitis flare-up. Fortunately, the flare-up only affected my left foot, but I was in major pain. Nothing I tried worked to bring me relief. I worried that without my ability to comfortably walk, the planned trip would be ruined.

That's when Olivia introduced me to Earthing Flipflops.

I never expected my grounders to bring me such happiness.

Since I started wearing my grounders, my pain from Plantar Fasciitis is minimal and more often completely gone, nothing debilitating or worrisome like before. I'm continually shocked by how much my situation improved after I started regularly wearing these new kicks.

During my trip, I walked around Las Vegas without any pain. The grounders kept me safe and sound; no problem walking all day with them on my feet!

EARTHING HAS CHANGED my life and the lives of many people I know. I have witnessed in myself and others the change that grounding can bring to one's quality of life. I love Clint for his remarkable discovery, and I will always be forever grateful to him and his life's work.

My love for the outdoors and all things natural runs deep, and grounding gives me the ability to enjoy more and more of it.[1]

---

1. Research References
    9. Classification of EEG Signal for Body Earthing Application 2018
    https://earthinginstitute.net/wp-content/uploads/2021/10/RahmanAl.EEG_
    for_Body-Earthing_Application-2018-1.pdf
    14. One-Hour Contact with the Earth's Surface (Grounding) Improves Inflammation and Blood Flow—A Randomized, Double-Blind, Pilot Study 2015
    www.scirp.org/Journal/PaperInformation.aspx?PaperID=58836
    15The Effect of Grounding the Human Body on Mood 2015

prx.sagepub.com/content/116/2/534.full.pdf+html

22. Emotional Stress, Heart Rate Variability, Grounding, and Improved Autonomic Tone: Clinical Applications 2011

https://earthinginstitute.net/wp-content/uploads/2016/07/Emotional-stress-study.pdf

30. The Biologic Effects of Grounding the Human Body During Sleep as Measured by Cortisol Levels and Subjective Reporting of Sleep, Pain, and Stress 2004

https://earthinginstitute.net/wp-content/uploads/2016/07/Cortisol-Study.pdf

41. The effects of grounding (earthing) on inflammation, the immune response, wound healing, and prevention and treatment of chronic inflammatory and autoimmune diseases.

https://pubmed.ncbi.nlm.nih.gov/25848315/

https://pubmed.ncbi.nlm.nih.gov/28987038/

42. Earthing: health implications of reconnecting the human body to the Earth's surface electrons.

https://pubmed.ncbi.nlm.nih.gov/22291721/

44. Electric Nutrition: The Surprising Health and Healing Benefits of Biological Grounding (Earthing).

46. The effect of grounding the human body on mood.

https://pubmed.ncbi.nlm.nih.gov/25748085/

52. The biologic effects of grounding the human body during sleep as measured by cortisol levels and subjective reporting of sleep, pain, and stress.

https://pubmed.ncbi.nlm.nih.gov/15650465/

12

LIFE AS WE KNOW IT

FIBROMYALGIA & PAIN

BILLIE RINEHART

*G*rowing up in the tropical forests of Panama, surrounded by lush trees, flowers, and animals all day, every day, connected me to something bigger than myself.

My mother, always outside in nature, took us to the beach and rivers. There, we ran barefoot. I remember the feeling of wellness and health these activities gave me.

Living that way brought me a connection I believe others must feel to understand, a relationship with grounding.

But even with this joy and connection, at some point, life veered in a different direction, and I left behind my outdoor adventures.

In hindsight, I believe that if I had never left my grounded connection, I could have saved myself from a lot of pain throughout my life. Instead, I grew disconnected, which left me open and vulnerable to pain.

As a young person, there were many opportunities to stay healthy —but I saw many who thought themselves invincible and often didn't take the best care of their bodies. As people age, if their bodies aren't properly cared for physically and mentally, their bodies change for the worse.

During my 64 years of knowledge of self-care, I continually relied on two things—diet and exercise—to create my health.

Still, even with a healthy life, after I turned 40, everything changed. Diet and exercise didn't offer the same support, and the unexpected occurred.

The chronic pain I saw in others found its way to me; I never expected to struggle with it myself.

Instead of restful nights, sleep became a trap of constant problems. In turn, my poor sleep caused numerous health disruptions and changed how I felt daily.

As time passed, issues with my hip, lower back, and feet developed. I thought, at first, these changes came from just getting older. The tightness I felt in my muscles made sense because they were all weight-bearing muscles used during daily activities such as walking or standing for long periods. Over the years, this same stiffness confined my movements, and I found myself indoors without any earth beneath my feet.

Eventually, having been diagnosed with fibromyalgia, I believed I had no choice other than poor health. Over the years, I dealt with the pain and the decline in health that accompanied this disease.

When the opportunity to use daily grounding techniques first arose, my painful hip made it difficult for me to do the exercises. The stiffness in the muscles of my hip made each movement painful.

Nowadays, though, my hip doesn't even bother me! Grounded exercise improved my ability to move around, and now I move without feeling pain or discomfort.

The grounding products I use positively changed my life so much so that when I found out my mother had fallen and couldn't move her arm because of the pain, I knew what I wanted to do.

I shared these Earthing products with my mother in Panama. I knew sending her one of the pillowcases would surely make a difference.

A strong woman, my mother never took pain medication for her ailments. Unfortunately, due to past trauma through medical negligence, Mother grew wary of doctors and refused to go no matter how much her children told her she needed a visit.

To add even more complications to her experience of this fall, her fall came during the first year of COVID, which increased her terror as she thought of going to the hospital where she surely would encounter the virus.

Thank goodness, the pillowcase I sent her did the trick. Mother went from being unable to move her arm to be able to move it freely and without pain!

Delighted with the results, my mother happily returned to her regular gardening routine, which keeps her planted in the earth.

Like me, many others agree that they feel better on the beach, with the sand between their toes, the mountains with the trees surrounding them, and the soil beneath their feet. They find that this connection dissolves away any feelings of depression or anxiety they experience while uprooted and disconnected from nature.

Human beings have a fundamental need to feel connected. The general sense of disconnection many people are experiencing today can be transformed through that connection I experienced all those years ago as a child.

I trust that by taking the time to reconnect to nature, others could find the same relief and health that I found.[1]

---

1. Research References
   9. Classification of EEG Signal for Body Earthing Application 2018
   https://earthinginstitute.net/wp-content/uploads/2021/10/RahmanAl.EEG_
   for_Body-Earthing_Application-2018-1.pdf
   14. One-Hour Contact with the Earth's Surface (Grounding) Improves Inflammation and Blood Flow—A Randomized, Double-Blind, Pilot Study 2015
   www.scirp.org/Journal/PaperInformation.aspx?PaperID=58836
   15The Effect of Grounding the Human Body on Mood 2015
   prx.sagepub.com/content/116/2/534.full.pdf+html
   22. Emotional Stress, Heart Rate Variability, Grounding, and Improved Autonomic Tone: Clinical Applications 2011
   https://earthinginstitute.net/wp-content/uploads/2016/07/Emotional-stress-study.pdf
   30. The Biologic Effects of Grounding the Human Body During Sleep as

Measured by Cortisol Levels and Subjective Reporting of Sleep, Pain, and Stress 2004

https://earthinginstitute.net/wp-content/uploads/2016/07/Cortisol-Study.pdf

41. The effects of grounding (earthing) on inflammation, the immune response, wound healing, and prevention and treatment of chronic inflammatory and autoimmune diseases.

https://pubmed.ncbi.nlm.nih.gov/25848315/

https://pubmed.ncbi.nlm.nih.gov/28987038/

42. Earthing: health implications of reconnecting the human body to the Earth's surface electrons.

https://pubmed.ncbi.nlm.nih.gov/22291721/

44. Electric Nutrition: The Surprising Health and Healing Benefits of Biological Grounding (Earthing).

46. The effect of grounding the human body on mood.

https://pubmed.ncbi.nlm.nih.gov/25748085/

52. The biologic effects of grounding the human body during sleep as measured by cortisol levels and subjective reporting of sleep, pain, and stress.

https://pubmed.ncbi.nlm.nih.gov/15650465/

13

BAD TO THE BONES

FIBROUS DYSPLASIA, SINUS, IRRITABLE BOWEL SYNDROME, & INFECTION

TERRIE GOSSARD FLINT

I have a rare bone disease called Fibrous Dysplasia. My disease weakens almost all the bones in my body. As my body tries to compensate for my bone weakness, the constant effort stresses my muscles, which become inflamed. In addition to my bone issue, my spine is twisted. A plate and screws were added to my left leg where I broke it several years ago.

My left shoulder needs to be replaced.

The muscles in my left arm greatly overcompensate for my bad shoulder so much that by nightfall I am almost in tears daily. My arm gets stuck at my side and is unable to function as the muscles just tangle up into huge knots. My husband massages the knots so I can move my arm to get undressed for bed.

So you really need to hear me when I say, "Grounding has changed my life."

My longtime friend, Sheri Rankin, told me of her involvement in something she thought could benefit me. Though she was still learning about it, she was anxious to educate me on the benefits.

"Grab five of your friends. We're going to give grounding a try."

"Grounding?" I queried.

"Grounding." She confirmed.

So, one Thursday at 10 a.m., I rounded up a handful of friends and met with Sheri. Everyone, including me, was skeptical as we sat down in chairs with those black mats under our feet and blankets over our laps. After Sheri connected us to some patches, she played a video explaining all the details.

The video introduced the concept, the benefits, how it helps your body, and the gentlemen we had to thank for coming up with the entire Earthing method.

Now, I have made a point of telling you that it was ten in the morning because one of the benefits of this treatment is sleeping better. And that morning, while I watched the video, snuggled in, and hooked up to grounding, I fell asleep!

I thought, "Oh, I'm just tired. It can't be the mat and blanket."

Then I felt a little pull on my arm, leg, and side. I dismissed those just as quickly, saying, "Can't be the treatment."

Even though the information made perfect sense, our little group remained skeptical that something this easy could do that much.

So, we decided to try it again.

We met the next week, and afterward, we all decided to give grounding a further try. Some of the ladies purchased the mats and some patches. Still skeptical, I went with the patches. It seemed like less of an investment and something easy just to push away if it didn't work in the end.

That first night, I felt something happen in my body.

That following day, my arm felt a little bit better.

My husband, who massaged my arm to get it to move, started showing interest. The condition of my arm persuaded him, and he wanted to try this grounding, too!

I called Sheri and asked for a pad for our bed and a pillowcase for my husband, thinking it might help with his bad neck pain.

We put the mat on our bed the day it arrived, and my husband used the case that night. We both felt a difference.

I felt that pull again. A slight pain arose in my side. Not a bad pain, but just like a little pulling discomfort.

I felt the muscles changing further in my bad arm.

My husband woke up in a sweat, feeling the grounded pillowcase working on his neck and back.

Over the next three months, our lives changed drastically.

My arm no longer bothers me daily. I can move it at will without pain and I don't need the extra massage from my husband.

My back feels so much better. I sleep well. I go to bed earlier and wake up before my alarm goes off. Each morning, I feel rested and more alert.

My husband spent a few nights away from home for work. He immediately noticed a difference. When he returned home, he couldn't wait to get into bed and get grounded to feel better. His neck and back pain that returned while traveling completely disappeared in a single night with his pillowcase.

For this reason, we take our grounding items with us on vacation because we refuse to be in pain if we don't have to for even one more day.

So much in my body has changed. I used to get sinus infections about three times a year, and they would be bad, and sometimes I would end up in the hospital. Well, that degree of infection stopped when I started grounding. I still get a sinus infection about once a year, but it is manageable.

I've lost some weight.

My irritable bowel syndrome is almost gone. I had so much trouble with that before grounding. I used to be constipated. My bathroom habits are regular now too.

Before getting my Earthing products, I had to watch everything I ate. I couldn't eat anything spicy or rich, or I'd be sick for the next couple of days. That's changed! I only remember one episode since I've been grounded.

Crazy...I know, but I feel 95% better since I've been grounded.

. . .

A FEW YEARS AGO, following surgery, I had a bad infection that wouldn't go away, and I felt awful. My husband brought me a small mat to the hospital. He put it under the case of my pillow and plugged it in.

I woke up with my pillowcase soaked through. Sure enough, my fever broke! It wasn't long before my infection passed, and I was able to come home.

It's amazing how much grounding has changed my life. I share the information with everyone I can. People think I must be selling it because I'm so passionate about it. I don't sell them; I just want everyone to feel as good as we do.

I am forever grateful to Sheri for sharing Earthing with my friends and me. My life changed for the better, and I know the whole world needs grounding, too. [1]

---

1. Research References
   9. Classification of EEG Signal for Body Earthing Application 2018
   https://earthinginstitute.net/wp-content/uploads/2021/10/RahmanAl.EEG_for_Body-Earthing_Application-2018-1.pdf
   14. One-Hour Contact with the Earth's Surface (Grounding) Improves Inflammation and Blood Flow—A Randomized, Double-Blind, Pilot Study 2015
   www.scirp.org/Journal/PaperInformation.aspx?PaperID=58836
   15The Effect of Grounding the Human Body on Mood 2015
   prx.sagepub.com/content/116/2/534.full.pdf+html
   22. Emotional Stress, Heart Rate Variability, Grounding, and Improved Autonomic Tone: Clinical Applications 2011
   https://earthinginstitute.net/wp-content/uploads/2016/07/Emotional-stress-study.pdf
   30. The Biologic Effects of Grounding the Human Body During Sleep as Measured by Cortisol Levels and Subjective Reporting of Sleep, Pain, and Stress 2004
   https://earthinginstitute.net/wp-content/uploads/2016/07/Cortisol-Study.pdf
   41. The effects of grounding (earthing) on inflammation, the immune response, wound healing, and prevention and treatment of chronic inflammatory and autoimmune diseases.
   https://pubmed.ncbi.nlm.nih.gov/25848315/
   42. Earthing: health implications of reconnecting the human body to the Earth's surface electrons.
   https://pubmed.ncbi.nlm.nih.gov/22291721/
   44. Electric Nutrition: The Surprising Health and Healing Benefits of Biological Grounding (Earthing).

https://pubmed.ncbi.nlm.nih.gov/28987038/

46. The effect of grounding the human body on mood.
https://pubmed.ncbi.nlm.nih.gov/25748085/

52. The biologic effects of grounding the human body during sleep as measured by cortisol levels and subjective reporting of sleep, pain, and stress.
https://pubmed.ncbi.nlm.nih.gov/15650465/

14

THE BIG C

CANCER, ATTITUDE, & ACHY JOINTS

STACY PLAZIAK

*A*fter my cancer treatment sessions, I felt tired and depressed. I found my normally positive attitude and my constant happy-go-lucky personality were harder and harder to maintain. Having always been a very positive person, I found it painful to be less than myself. I resisted accepting that the drastic changes I experienced in my mood and attitude were permanent.

Seeing myself fade further and further into the background depressed me.

WHEN I BOUGHT A GROUNDING CHAIR, right away I noticed a change. I remember first sitting down. It was one of those "hmm" thoughts, like, "Okay, hmm."

I put my feet on the pad and within five to ten minutes the tingling sensation that started in my feet moved up to my bad knee, where it was really intense, and traveled up through my body and to the top of my head until my entire body just tingled.

Grounding helped my body feel better.

Grounding brought changes to my mental state.

Because my emotions changed, I recognized more of myself. Because the inflammation was reduced, I felt less pain. Without the distraction of pain, it was easier to be me. My attitude and thoughts changed. I found it easier to focus on my healing.

EVERY DOCTOR, including my phenomenal doctor, recognizes the common side effect of swelling that comes with cancer treatments. This vascular reaction or lymph issue causes an increase in the fluid of the cells to leak into the layers of the skin, resulting in swelling.

It is not an exaggeration to say that a LOT of swelling is expected.

To my doctor's astonishment, my body swelled very little.

In addition to the chemo treatment, within two days I'd have to give myself a shot in my stomach. The medicine I injected was unbelievably painful. It made my bones ache something fierce.

I couldn't lie down.

I couldn't stand up.

Everything hurt. I was so incredibly uncomfortable.

To help with this discomfort, for the first week after each one of my chemo treatments I slept in my grounding chair. It was the only thing that helped me endure the six months of treatment.

THE TIME CAME for the surgery to remove what was left of the cancer cells.

At my post-op appointment, my surgeon looked at me in disbelief and shared, "Wow, I just have to say, usually when we go in to remove a mass, there is a shell of where cancer used to be. But not with you. Yours is completely gone. The only indication you even had a previous mass was a small indentation in the tissue."

The doctors, the surgeon, my family, and I were all shocked.

The doctor was so excited about the chemo and how well it had worked. With her focus and faith in Western Medicine, my doctor only smiled when I told her about the support grounding gave me. I often wonder if her beliefs allow her to consider what I know to be true.

REMEMBER, I said I had a bad knee and that when the grounding tingles traveled to my knee the feeling was really intense? Here's why. I played basketball in high school. I tore a ligament in that knee and it just never healed properly.

For years I had flare-ups. I suffered from debilitating nerve pain that sometimes took me out of my daily routine for hours. To help with this pain, I had reconstructive surgery. Unfortunately, after the surgery, my knee was never the same. Instead, it remained swollen and in a constant state of inflammation. Grounding helped me live with this bum body part for years until I finally got the courage to try another surgery, a complete replacement, that fixed the issue. Besides grounding me, it's the best thing I ever did.

I USE the sheets and the pillowcases every night. On the rare occasion that I miss a night of being grounded, my joints ache. My hands and body feel stiff and uncomfortable. Because of these obvious changes, I use Earthing products religiously.

Now that I am much more aware of this much-needed practice, I also go barefoot a lot. This is a gift I give myself as grounding has changed my perspective on the different types of healing the world has to offer. I feel this natural medicine is my best life insurance policy.

When I am grounded, I feel that my risk of getting cancer, or any other disease, drastically decreases. More than just a belief I picked up, there is proof. Studies show time and time again that many of the diseases and causes of pain we endure are caused by inflammation in our bodies. Science understands that grounding drastically reduces inflammation.

This extra layer of comfort, my grounding practice, offered me a new lease on life.

It isn't just the big life-changing differences that I am grateful for. It is the return of a quality of life I never expected could be possible. My daughter is getting married soon, and because I have this support, I am so excited about the future. I am excited about the possibility of grandchildren. Before grounding, I don't think I would have ever thought it possible to feel good and have enough energy to be an active grandmother.

The support Earthing brought to my life gave me hope, and I love being alive!

I love living![1]

---

1. Research References

    9. Classification of EEG Signal for Body Earthing Application 2018
    https://earthinginstitute.net/wp-content/uploads/2021/10/RahmanAl.EEG_ for_Body-Earthing_Application-2018-1.pdf
    14. One-Hour Contact with the Earth's Surface (Grounding) Improves Inflammation and Blood Flow—A Randomized, Double-Blind, Pilot Study 2015
    www.scirp.org/Journal/PaperInformation.aspx?PaperID=58836
    15The Effect of Grounding the Human Body on Mood 2015
    prx.sagepub.com/content/116/2/534.full.pdf+html
    22. Emotional Stress, Heart Rate Variability, Grounding, and Improved Autonomic Tone: Clinical Applications 2011
    https://earthinginstitute.net/wp-content/uploads/2016/07/Emotional-stress-study.pdf
    30. The Biologic Effects of Grounding the Human Body During Sleep as Measured by Cortisol Levels and Subjective Reporting of Sleep, Pain, and Stress 2004
    https://earthinginstitute.net/wp-content/uploads/2016/07/Cortisol-Study.pdf
    41. The effects of grounding (earthing) on inflammation, the immune response, wound healing, and prevention and treatment of chronic inflammatory and autoimmune diseases.
    https://pubmed.ncbi.nlm.nih.gov/25848315/
    https://pubmed.ncbi.nlm.nih.gov/28987038/
    42. Earthing: health implications of reconnecting the human body to the Earth's surface electrons.
    https://pubmed.ncbi.nlm.nih.gov/22291721/
    44. Electric Nutrition: The Surprising Health and Healing Benefits of Biological Grounding (Earthing).
    46. The effect of grounding the human body on mood.
    https://pubmed.ncbi.nlm.nih.gov/25748085/

52. The biologic effects of grounding the human body during sleep as measured by cortisol levels and subjective reporting of sleep, pain, and stress. https://pubmed.ncbi.nlm.nih.gov/15650465/

15

AGAINST THE GRAIN

INJURY FROM FALLS & CHRONIC PAIN

TERESA PODGORSKI

I **Am a Physician Assistant**
I am a physician assistant with firsthand knowledge of the amazing power we have in our Western medical treatments.

But, even with these broad strokes that support our medical knowledge, I have witnessed gaps and limits within what traditional medicine can achieve.

Many physicians are skeptical of methods and modalities that are unfamiliar to them, those that are currently considered untraditional, and that they view as fringe science. They are against using products or concepts like grounding in their practice of medicine and consider those who do incorporate grounding or other methods of healing to be "odd" or quacks.

IN MY EXPERIENCE, those who truly believe there is balance in all things find themselves open to the implementation of western medicine and grounding together. The difference the combination of these practices makes in people's lives is astounding.

I AM an Advocate

I am a huge advocate for grounding, and I use it every day.

Grounding has changed my life, and I have been a personal witness to the lives around me that it has changed. I even named one of my four dogs Clinton, as a reminder that I am forever grateful to Clint Ober for his ingenuity, perseverance, and his discovery of Earthing.

Even with all this faith and trust in my personal life based on first-hand experiences, I find that my patients are often very much non-believers when it comes to other methods of healing.

Instead of selling people on the idea that their bodies need to be healed, I let them experience it themselves. I suggest to these skeptics that they sit outside in a chair with their feet in the grass. If they do that every day for an hour and nothing changes and nothing feels different in their bodies, then they've got me!

Most folks look at me like I am crazy, sharing, "There is no way that something so simple can help." I offer just a smile and encourage them to give it a try.

"It can't hurt, and it's free."

After trying grounding for an hour with no other effort, when they realize they feel better in no time flat they're hooked!

My favorite thing is seeing someone's face light up after they achieve self-healing. There isn't anything more rewarding.

I CARE for Others

In 2015, my mom had a nasty fall that resulted in a very severe shoulder injury. The doctors put a plate with six screws in and a bone graft to keep her in one piece. It was a very big operation. What the doctors didn't know going into the surgery was that my mom could not take pain medication. Heavy painkillers cause her to hallucinate and get very sick.

For me, as a healthcare provider, seeing the severity of her injury and knowing she couldn't take pain medication, the entire ordeal was terrifying. I had worried endlessly about how she could get through this recovery using just Tylenol.

Fortunately, Clint gave me all the grounding products she needed for a speedy recovery. Throughout her recovery, the only time she was even remotely comfortable was when she was grounded.

Grounding was the sole solution.

I will forever be grateful to Clint for his discovery and friendship.

Grounding got my mother through the after-surgery experience and on the road to recovery.

I Have Pain

I have chronic pain, and grounding gives me the ability to function and live.

In 2017, I underwent surgery for carpal tunnel and cubital tunnel at the same time. They operated on my wrist and my elbow to release the nerves and put an end to my years of pain and inflammation.

My surgeon warned me that recovery would be tough and quite painful. I was never a fan of taking heavy pain medications and opted to go the same route as my mother and only use Tylenol for my recovery. As long as I stayed grounded, I was fine and there was no pain.

I also have degenerative disc disease, which is a condition that can cause pain and inflammation in my back. For many people, staying active and keeping the back strong is the best way to prevent or manage symptoms.

However, when flare-ups occur, it can be difficult to stay active. That's where a grounding chair comes into play for me. Sitting in a grounding chair helps to alleviate pain and inflammation and can make it easier to get through a flare-up.

In addition to chiropractic care, grounding is the most effective way for me to handle flare-ups. It allows me the ability to still hike and stay active when I otherwise would be down for days in agony.

I LOVINGLY ACCEPT Mother Earth

Consider this, water and air are necessary for survival. These are provided for us by Mother Earth. As humans, why would we think that Mother Earth only offers us these two things to aid in our survival?

We accept freely and without question that we need air and water. Take a leap of faith and see how much more Mother Earth can provide for you. She is powerful, just as our connection to her is powerful.

My wish for humanity is that we take care of the earth, take care of her so that she can continue to take care of us.[1]

---

1. Research References
   9. Classification of EEG Signal for Body Earthing Application 2018
   https://earthinginstitute.net/wp-content/uploads/2021/10/RahmanAl.EEG_for_Body-Earthing_Application-2018-1.pdf
   14. One-Hour Contact with the Earth's Surface (Grounding) Improves Inflammation and Blood Flow—A Randomized, Double-Blind, Pilot Study 2015
   www.scirp.org/Journal/PaperInformation.aspx?PaperID=58836
   15The Effect of Grounding the Human Body on Mood 2015
   prx.sagepub.com/content/116/2/534.full.pdf+html
   22. Emotional Stress, Heart Rate Variability, Grounding, and Improved Autonomic Tone: Clinical Applications 2011
   https://earthinginstitute.net/wp-content/uploads/2016/07/Emotional-stress-study.pdf
   30. The Biologic Effects of Grounding the Human Body During Sleep as Measured by Cortisol Levels and Subjective Reporting of Sleep, Pain, and Stress 2004
   https://earthinginstitute.net/wp-content/uploads/2016/07/Cortisol-Study.pdf
   41. The effects of grounding (earthing) on inflammation, the immune response, wound healing, and prevention and treatment of chronic inflammatory and autoimmune diseases.
   https://pubmed.ncbi.nlm.nih.gov/25848315/
   https://pubmed.ncbi.nlm.nih.gov/28987038/
   42. Earthing: health implications of reconnecting the human body to the Earth's surface electrons.
   https://pubmed.ncbi.nlm.nih.gov/22291721/

44. Electric Nutrition: The Surprising Health and Healing Benefits of Biological Grounding (Earthing).

46. The effect of grounding the human body on mood.
https://pubmed.ncbi.nlm.nih.gov/25748085/

52. The biologic effects of grounding the human body during sleep as measured by cortisol levels and subjective reporting of sleep, pain, and stress.
https://pubmed.ncbi.nlm.nih.gov/15650465/

16

NO WAY BACK

TRANSVERSE MYELITIS, PARALYSIS, & INFLAMMATION

JULIENNE DALLARA

*A*s a performer, dancer, singer, and actress, I lived a very mobile and active life. Even my hobbies kept me active, as I loved being outdoors, hiking mountains in Alaska, and swimming in the ocean around Hawaii.

My life of activity delivered everything to me until a day in 1997 when I woke up to find myself completely paralyzed.

My diagnosis is an incurable disease called transverse myelitis.

What a shock!

To say it was a harsh change, in reality, would be an understatement. My entire world permanently changed overnight.

Some of the things that instantly ended for me included:

- trips to the beach where I put my toes in the sand
- tikes to the top of a mountain to feel the brisk air around me
- my constant connection to the earth and her wonders
- my performance career and dancing

- a life of freedom and fluidity
- the care I gave my young children—ages 3 years old, and 7 months

So much was completely and instantly taken away from me.

BUT AS ONE DOES, I considered my choice. I could adapt and make the best of it or I could suffer. I chose to adapt. Still alive, I was going to make the best of it.

One of my first steps toward freedom brought me to apply with a charity for a handicap-accessible van.

The day I went to pick up my van, the company offered me a job on the spot. I took a breath and embraced the idea that the universe knew exactly what I needed. Slowly, the job brought a blessing of normalcy back to my life and I spent the next 15 years selling handicap-accessible vehicles. I loved being able to work in such a rewarding career. My ability to help those in need of my support was a huge plus!

The day came when I got an email from the Abilities Expo. They wanted me to interview for a spot on their team. Abilities Expo is the premiere event for the disabled community. For three days, everyone gets to see and try the latest products and services, cutting-edge tech, information-packed workshops, adaptive activities, and so much more.

Abilities Expo had a wish list of three people, and I was on it! The job was mine, and fortunately, through that job, I found out about grounding.

I met the Earthing team at one of the expos where I tried the chair. It was such a surreal experience that when I was offered the mat for my bed, I eagerly accepted.

In just one night, the remarkable reduction of inflammation in my feet was life-changing. The difference was so noticeable that even my husband, ever the cynic, conceded to the reality of this amazing change and turned the mat so that we could both have our feet on it at night.

That was years ago, and grounding continues to play a part in both of our lives. Because of the huge difference in using both the grounding mat and the pillowcase made for us, we will never be without these amazing products. It's wonderful to have my feet grounded, and my neck resting on the pillow. The sensation of being connected to Earth and her power is one I never expected to have again in my life.

Traveling in the past brought me the typical stress that it does for everyone. While away from home, my sleep is so much more restless. I lose that settled feeling to which I am accustomed. The feeling of separation I have when ungrounded leaves me thinking so many things are just not right. Thanks to Earthing products, this unsettled feeling during travel is no longer part of my life.

I believe we are meant to be connected to Mother Earth. We are meant to feel the energy she gives us, her continued fuel of support flowing through us.

She heals us.

Those who are wheelchair-bound don't get to experience the Earth like everyone else. My capacity to embrace these amazing Earthing products while in a wheelchair brings an entirely new dimension to my life. I am truly grateful for the ability to ground myself even as a differently-abled person.

Earthing brought Mother Earth into my home, and I will forever be grateful. [1]

---

1. Research References
   9. Classification of EEG Signal for Body Earthing Application 2018
   https://earthinginstitute.net/wp-content/uploads/2021/10/RahmanAl.EEG_
   for_Body-Earthing_Application-2018-1.pdf
   14. One-Hour Contact with the Earth's Surface (Grounding) Improves Inflammation and Blood Flow—A Randomized, Double-Blind, Pilot Study 2015
   www.scirp.org/Journal/PaperInformation.aspx?PaperID=58836
   15The Effect of Grounding the Human Body on Mood 2015
   prx.sagepub.com/content/116/2/534.full.pdf+html

22. Emotional Stress, Heart Rate Variability, Grounding, and Improved Autonomic Tone: Clinical Applications 2011

https://earthinginstitute.net/wp-content/uploads/2016/07/Emotional-stress-
study.pdf

30. The Biologic Effects of Grounding the Human Body During Sleep as
Measured by Cortisol Levels and Subjective Reporting of Sleep, Pain, and
Stress 2004

https://earthinginstitute.net/wp-content/uploads/2016/07/Cortisol-Study.pdf

41. The effects of grounding (earthing) on inflammation, the immune response,
wound healing, and prevention and treatment of chronic inflammatory and
autoimmune diseases.

https://pubmed.ncbi.nlm.nih.gov/25848315/

https://pubmed.ncbi.nlm.nih.gov/28987038/

42. Earthing: health implications of reconnecting the human body to the Earth's
surface electrons.

https://pubmed.ncbi.nlm.nih.gov/22291721/

44. Electric Nutrition: The Surprising Health and Healing Benefits of Biological
Grounding (Earthing).

46. The effect of grounding the human body on mood.

https://pubmed.ncbi.nlm.nih.gov/25748085/

52. The biologic effects of grounding the human body during sleep as measured
by cortisol levels and subjective reporting of sleep, pain, and stress.

https://pubmed.ncbi.nlm.nih.gov/15650465/

17

TAKE A SEAT, PLEASE

INCREASED HEALTH, QUALITY OF LIFE, CENTERED, GROUNDED, & REDUCED ANXIETY

GABRIELLE FORLEO

J'm the number one all-time salesperson at the Chopra Center for Wellbeing. I've worked with Deepak for sixteen years and have the privilege of being the lead yoga instructor at the company's retreats. In addition to my work at the Chopra Center, I run my own business. I am a money mindset coach for female entrepreneurs.

With my credentials, you might be surprised to know that I was initially totally skeptical about grounding. You see, Deepak does a lot of kooky things, and not all of them initially make sense.

I noticed the grounding chair for at least three of our Chopra events and never even tried it. Skeptical, the products held no interest for me.

The first time I got in the chair came just before going on stage to speak in front of 500 people. I thought to myself, "Now is as good a time as any to just try out these kooky chairs."

Never before in my life had I felt so good and so grounded!

All I did was sit down in the chair and engage zero gravity and I was blown away. After a brief sit, I proceeded to go on stage and kill it with an awesome presentation. During the presentation, I noticed the difference the chair made—I felt more present and really calm.

Such an incredible change. I became immediately obsessed.

I bought everyone in my family a grounding mat.

I became the person at Chopra retreats who would be like, "You have to go sit in this chair."

I also purchased the mat for my partner, who at the time had sleep apnea. Six years later, not one recurrence of his apnea episodes. The mat is magic!

I turned my mom and stepmom on too, and at first, they were both skeptical. They claimed that they didn't notice any changes, but once they stopped using the product, they definitely noticed what was missing and went back to using their Earthing tool.

I find it so interesting that some people appear not to notice the effects until they have missed a night of sleeping on the mat. Others notice the effects right away. Every unique experience brings up more interest in the process for me.

I've been Earthing for about nine years. I can't express enough how much healthier I am. I am more centered and grounded and I feel less anxious. My overall quality of life has improved tenfold, and I recommend the products to anyone who will listen.

My only regret is that I wish I had started down this path far earlier without the experience of being skeptical and closed off. Now, I absolutely recommend everyone give Earthing a try.

What is it going to hurt?

Nothing.

It's the easiest, most beautiful healing modality in the entire world.[1]

---

1. Research References
   6. The Effects of Grounding (Earthing) on Bodyworkers' Pain and Overall Quality of Life: A randomized Controlled Trial 2019
      https://www.sciencedirect.com/science/article/pii/S1550830718302519
   9. Classification of EEG Signal for Body Earthing Application 2018
      https://earthinginstitute.net/wp-content/uploads/2021/10/RahmanAl.EEG_for_Body-Earthing_Application-2018-1.pdf

13. Grounding After Moderate Eccentric Contractions Reduces Muscle Damage 2015

https://www.dovepress.com/articles.php?article_id=2377114.   One-Hour Contact with the Earth's Surface (Grounding) Improves Inflammation and Blood Flow—A Randomized, Double-Blind, Pilot Study 2015

www.scirp.org/Journal/PaperInformation.aspx?PaperID=58836

15The Effect of Grounding the Human Body on Mood 2015

prx.sagepub.com/content/116/2/534.full.pdf+html

16. Grounding the Human Body during Yoga Exercise with a Grounded Yoga Mat Reduces Blood Viscosity 2015

http://www.scirp.org/Journal/PaperInformation.aspx?PaperID=55445#.VSa19_nF_7A

22. Emotional Stress, Heart Rate Variability, Grounding, and Improved Autonomic Tone: Clinical Applications 2011

https://earthinginstitute.net/wp-content/uploads/2016/07/Emotional-stress-study.pdf

30. The Biologic Effects of Grounding the Human Body During Sleep as Measured by Cortisol Levels and Subjective Reporting of Sleep, Pain, and Stress 2004

https://earthinginstitute.net/wp-content/uploads/2016/07/Cortisol-Study.pdf

42. Earthing: health implications of reconnecting the human body to the Earth's surface electrons.

https://pubmed.ncbi.nlm.nih.gov/22291721/

43. The Effects of Grounding (Earthing) on Bodyworkers' Pain and Overall Quality of Life: A Randomized Controlled Trial.

https://pubmed.ncbi.nlm.nih.gov/30448083/

46. The effect of grounding the human body on mood.

https://pubmed.ncbi.nlm.nih.gov/25748085/

48. Grounding after moderate eccentric contractions reduces muscle damage.

https://pubmed.ncbi.nlm.nih.gov/26443876/

52. The biologic effects of grounding the human body during sleep as measured by cortisol levels and subjective reporting of sleep, pain, and stress.

https://pubmed.ncbi.nlm.nih.gov/15650465/

18

FOR GINNY'S SAKE, COMFORT FIRST

PAIN RELIEF, SLEEP, & CANINE COMFORT

EIKE CAPELLE

A couple of years ago, my husband and I watched The Earthing Movie. Immediately, I investigated the possibility of adding grounding measures to our lives.

I always felt most comfortable when I walked barefoot, so the science made sense to me. I felt more relaxed and at peace when in the water. And the beach, with my toesies stuck in the sand, that's the absolute best.

Even during the harsh Wisconsin winters, if even for only a few minutes, I took breaks to sneak out barefoot for the jolt it gives me as I connect to the frozen earth.

Knowing that both my husband and I were dealing with plenty of health issues related to inflammation, I couldn't place my order for the mattress grounding sheets fast enough.

While using the products, I noticed small, slight changes. See, I had a heck of a time sleeping, and I noticed that I felt a bit more rested and less anxious. I find it comforting to rest my legs on the sheets and know that I can trust in the well-documented science made available by Clint Ober and his team. Earthing makes me feel good and I know that my body is benefiting from the connection.

My husband, bless his heart, is not a man who embraces change with his arms wide open. He didn't really care for the sheets, and in all fairness, he wasn't willing to give it a good try. More of a man who seeks instant gratification, he decided they weren't for him, and he moved the grounding sheet to our guest bedroom for me to use on my own when needed.

Over time, I noticed our dog Ginny, a sixty-pound black Golden retriever mix, often made herself quite comfortable on the modified guest bed. Diagnosed with Cushing's disease, Ginny dealt with extreme panting. At times she had a hard time regulating her body temperature. She seemed less restless on the sheet and finally, she claimed it as her own.

Before Ginny took over the grounding sheet, she would hide in the basement on the concrete floor in the dark corners. After she began using the sheet, lying outside on the patio or on the grass became her preferred way to rest. The moment she comes inside from the backyard, it is either the grounded bed or her cooling gel pad. I have even seen her with half of her body on both.

For Ginny's sake, we never leave home without her sheet, which we even take camping with us for our sweet Ginny to lie on.

Animals are so much smarter than us. It makes total sense to me that my dog does what is best for her.

I will be forever grateful for the invention of these great products. I share the science of Earthing with anyone who wants to hear about it and even those who might not. I will forever praise the day Clint Ober took his first barefoot walk on this earth and made the essential and life-changing discovery of Earthing.

Now, all we need is for Clint Ober and his team to come out with a grounded dog bed with a removable, washable cover.[1]

---

1. Research References
    9. Classification of EEG Signal for Body Earthing Application 2018

https://earthinginstitute.net/wp-content/uploads/2021/10/RahmanAl.EEG_
for_Body-Earthing_Application-2018-1.pdf

14. One-Hour Contact with the Earth's Surface (Grounding) Improves Inflammation and Blood Flow—A Randomized, Double-Blind, Pilot Study 2015
www.scirp.org/Journal/PaperInformation.aspx?PaperID=58836
15The Effect of Grounding the Human Body on Mood 2015
prx.sagepub.com/content/116/2/534.full.pdf+html

22. Emotional Stress, Heart Rate Variability, Grounding, and Improved Autonomic Tone: Clinical Applications 2011
https://earthinginstitute.net/wp-content/uploads/2016/07/Emotional-stress-
study.pdf

30. The Biologic Effects of Grounding the Human Body During Sleep as
Measured by Cortisol Levels and Subjective Reporting of Sleep, Pain, and
Stress 2004
https://earthinginstitute.net/wp-content/uploads/2016/07/Cortisol-Study.pdf

41. The effects of grounding (earthing) on inflammation, the immune response,
wound healing, and prevention and treatment of chronic inflammatory and
autoimmune diseases.
https://pubmed.ncbi.nlm.nih.gov/25848315/
https://pubmed.ncbi.nlm.nih.gov/28987038/

42. Earthing: health implications of reconnecting the human body to the Earth's
surface electrons.
https://pubmed.ncbi.nlm.nih.gov/22291721/

44. Electric Nutrition: The Surprising Health and Healing Benefits of Biological
Grounding (Earthing).

46. The effect of grounding the human body on mood.
https://pubmed.ncbi.nlm.nih.gov/25748085/

52. The biologic effects of grounding the human body during sleep as measured
by cortisol levels and subjective reporting of sleep, pain, and stress.
https://pubmed.ncbi.nlm.nih.gov/15650465/

19

A TICKING TIME BOMB

HEMORRHAGING OF THE ESOPHAGEAL AND STOMACH VARICES, CIRRHOSIS OF THE LIVER, & HEPATITIS C

JANNA SAAVEDRA

Early one morning, I woke feeling a slight stomachache and headed to the guest bathroom, expecting to be sick. I had no idea a time bomb was about to explode inside me.

What came up was bright red, and it just kept coming up. My nightmarish scream that ensued woke my husband, who bore witness to this horrific event.

Seeing at least a liter of blood, he wanted to call for an ambulance.

Knowing what I must look like and the amount of blood on my sleepwear, I chose to take a shower before allowing him to drive me to the Emergency Room.

I HAD ALREADY BEGUN the first steps toward healing my alcoholism. I started the process of self-reflection. In addition, so I could sleep and feel better after my routine drinking bouts, I used Earthing products.

As an alcoholic who just loved to drink, I was happy to celebrate my 50th birthday. Coming from a hard beginning in life, the thought of 50 seemed unattainable.

Still, even with my history and the effort I had made to change, I was surprised when the time bomb, which I wanted to avoid, went off inside me.

OUR HOUSE WAS ONLY five miles from a small hospital, so the drive was short. Once there, I was seen rather quickly and immediately transported by ambulance to a much larger hospital.

There, they ran all labs known to mankind and put me into an MRI to confirm their diagnosis of hemorrhaging of the esophageal varices; these are what was bleeding out.

To top things off, my diagnosis included cirrhosis of the liver and additional varices in my stomach. I also had Hepatitis C, which went untreated for years.

The doctors urgently put me on medication, and the hospital released me with a no-drinking alcohol order and encouraged me to follow up with their gastroenterologist for surgery on the varices.

WITHOUT ANY INSURANCE, I had not been to a doctor in years. The main course of action was to find a primary care physician and learn what steps to take to get my health back to normal.

My new doctor laid out the plan. The steps included a liver transplant as the endgame. She explained we had a lot to accomplish to get me on the list. The first items were to stop drinking and cure my Hepatitis C.

After a month or two of fighting the system, my doctor got the approval for a new hepatitis drug. The drug was very expensive, but with the help and support of my family, it was purchased.

Thankfully, my fear of death seems to have delivered me from the urge to drink. I have not had a drink in seven months. I believe I will never have another drink for the rest of my life.

As I shared before, I was already using Earthing products. Upon hearing of my situation, Clint Ober advised me to ground my liver every night by placing the patches on the skin directly above the organ and sleep with them in place.

In addition to the patches, I also sleep on a grounded Earthing Sleep Mat and an Earthing Pillow Cover.

The final change I made is to take good care of myself with what I eat and drink.

As ADVISED, I used the Earthing patches every night until I fully recovered. I did this and continue to do so to this day.

My labs were taken after ten weeks of this focused grounding. The results that came back showed that Hepatitis C was no longer a problem. More importantly, my kidneys were working.

The detail that totally surprised my doctor was that my liver had recovered and was working as well. With all my numbers in the normal range, my liver was on the mend.

I can't explain how the act of connecting to the earth helped to heal my body. I can share that as soon as I ground, I instantly feel the pain and stress drain from my body. A soothing calm washes over me, supported by Earth's healing energy.

The Mother Earth Effect of grounding is real and because of it, I am looking forward to turning 51 with a new, well-grounded outlook on life!

HOME ON THE RANGE

ADRENAL FATIGUE

CLINT OBER

*T*he Perception

Picture a young Clint, his image pulled straight out of an old Hollywood Western movie, set tall atop a horse while he rides through the vast fields and pastures herding the family's cattle. Wherever they roamed, he roamed, with his cowboy hat dipped ever so slightly down in front to cut the glint of the sun from his eyes.

This old-fashioned imagery goes right to the heart of Clint's character and upbringing.

Clint spent his childhood on the family's cattle ranch near a Native American community. While he lived in the camaraderie of these peaceful people, he formed a relationship with nature's essential beauty and knowledge. He connected to the earth and its elements. He developed a natural, uncluttered way of viewing life and the world around him.

Often, when he embraced the rich culture of the Native American communities, he found moments of clarity. Their lifestyle influenced him, and he learned to see things in natural and magical ways.

. . .

As a rancher, Clint took his duties seriously; he was the keeper of the herd, responsible for their wellbeing. If one member gets sick, he goes through his checklist to safeguard the cattle and keep the rest of them well.

One of the tell-tale signs of a sick cow was a glassy-eyed stare. When found, Clint accompanied the sick animal to a holding corral, then rode along the entire pasture to investigate what caused the illness.

His checklist included such considerations:

- *Did the cow get a hold of weeds in the pasture and eat them?*
- *Was the PH balance of the water safe for drinking?*
- *Could the water upstream be poisoned or toxic?*

Often, it took hours to uncover the cause of the cow's illness, which he considered time well spent. He knew the importance of discovering the root cause of their illness. Treating their symptoms just wasn't enough.

One year, the ranch suffered an infestation of jackrabbits. The field glistened like water with so many pairs of shiny critter eyes.

Clint quietly observed the field full of rabbits as a coyote approached to hunt them. The predator sneaked up on its prey, and as the rabbit sensed the danger, its ears perked up. As the carnivore readied for the attack, the rabbit sprang into action.

The chase was on!

With one eye on the coyote and one in front to watch the terrain, the jackrabbit zig-zagged across the field. Clint followed what he considered to be a beautiful site and admired how the rabbit glided through the air effortlessly.

The coyote continued to run after its meal, but it was no match for the speedy creature, which dodged and veered in different directions.

The predator pressed on for a good while but eventually gave up in exhaustion. Clint chuckled as the rabbit claimed its victory.

Then, to his surprise, the hare ran a short distance from the exhausted coyote, stopped, and trembled.

Clint watched as the critter trembled for a moment longer, took a breath, and continued like nothing even happened, the chase already a memory.

Surprised and intrigued, he considered the rabbit's ability to shake off the chase, return to a peaceful state, and continue completely unencumbered after such a close call with death.

Eventually, after some consideration, Clint concluded that the rabbit discharged its stress into the ground. Through its violent shaking, it released the stress-filled hormones and returned to homeostasis, completely trauma free and without any burden.

His comprehension of the rabbit's release led Clint to coin the term "Earthing." Now commonly used in daily life, Earthing is the process by which the instantaneous discharge of electrical energy transfers these charges directly to the earth through contact.

THE PROBLEM

For years, Clint asked people how their illnesses came to be. Nearly every time, the answer came back the same, "I have no idea. It just showed up."

They often continued to share details of their lives, each telling him about their trials and the losses they experienced, as if the incidents were responsible for and defined their disease or illness.

Yet, Clint observed that the person sharing their story drew no direct parallels, while he saw the cause-and-effect impact of their trauma, fear, depression, loneliness, and more.

In 2011, Clint encountered a woman diagnosed with Multiple Sclerosis living a life of constant pain and stress, and who remained bedridden. When he first met her, he asked, as always, "Do you know what caused the MS to manifest?"

The woman had no idea.

For her, the disease dropped into her lap and continued to get worse.

She then told Clint her tale of woe. In 2008, three years before their meeting, she lost her job and home. She lived in a constant state of disappointment. Because of her distressed state, her body produced an elevated level of cortisol, which remained in her system without release.

The constant flow of this increased hormone in her body repeatedly activated her sympathetic nervous system. This activation causes constriction in blood flow. When this happens, the parasympathetic nervous system typically releases hormones to reduce and calm down the overactive sympathetic nervous system.

However, due to her persistent psychological unrest, the woman remained in a fight-or-flight state, which ensured and continued her extremely high cortisol level.

Additionally, unable to come out of fight-or-flight mode, she overworked her adrenals, which led to adrenal fatigue. She found herself with little or no energy.

Her daily experience of exhausted adrenals and her low level of cortisol, which she created by the constant influx of other stress-reducing hormones, made it harder for her to get out of bed. Her fatigue and exhaustion, in turn, caused more unrest as she could not fix her situation.

The debilitating process was a self-feeding loop and the cycle saw no end.

Clint saw that the woman must limit her exposure to coyotes; rather, she needed to reduce her stressors. She needed to get her out of flight-or-fight and reduce the hormones that kept her system on guard. Like the jackrabbit, her body craved Earthing.

If she could do that, she could get her life back.

THE PERFECTION

The constant exposure to the stories of others helped Clint begin to form a complete picture of the impact Earthing would have if put to good use.

He recalled seeing on TV the idea, "An apple a day keeps the doctor away."

Back then, people lived with this popular preventative and straightforward method of self-care.

In the early 1970s, the conversation shifted from prevention to intervention. The new mindset became, "Oh, don't worry about taking care of your health—once you're old, they'll have a cure for everything."

The general experience moved from self-grown, fresh seasonal food, where we relied on natural eating, to instant access to everything: food, entertainment, and more. The behavior of allowing our bodies and our minds to rely on nature came to an end, which eventually left more people sick than ever before, including Clint.

Clint retired from the cable industry at the age of fifty due to an abscessed liver. His condition, which required surgery, nearly killed him.

While lying in bed following his surgery, he looked past his feet to see his large wall hanging—a hand-painted picture by a famous western artist. In the painting, two small images can be seen of riders on horses.

The way he saw it, these riders connected to their surroundings using their hearts, bodies, and minds.

Reminded of his days back on the ranch, Clint returned to a feeling of oneness and equality. While only a small piece of the picture, the riders were a united part of the scenery and equal to their environment.

As he considered how close to death he had come and that the surgery he needed for his liver nearly killed him, he shifted internally and became a different person. He knew he must dump the current, artificial environment. He decided to focus his time and energy on ways that returned him to a more natural, cohesive environment.

Once Clint started his healing journey, he gave up everything that financially burdened him. Fighting for these burdens cost him his health and he realized, in comparison, that he didn't want any of them.

Clint's priority became one of *"better to give than to take,"* a new direction for him that he didn't have before his surgery.

As he chose to step into his spirituality, this earthy person popped out.

He explored this open connection to his renewed reality with RV travel. For four years, he connected with pine trees, the outdoors, mountains, and more. With fresh eyes, he witnessed the sky as a vibrant blue, the pine needles a more vibrant green, and everything in sight grew brighter.

At the time, Clint didn't know what had changed. He continued to pursue his feelings and his need to reawaken the more natural part of himself.

ONE EVENING, while watching the sunset in Key Largo, Florida, an irresistible desire overcame him. At first, he found it hard to pinpoint, only aware that the pressing emotion overwhelmed him and drew all his attention. Eventually, he relaxed enough and accepted the message spoken directly to him by Earth.

The powerful energy told him, *"Become an opposite charge."* Unsure of what it meant, he pulled out a pen and paper and wrote it down.

He continued to sit in quiet contemplation until the energy spoke again, *"Status quo is the enemy."*

He quickly wrote down this message, still unsure where either statement might take him.

After a few days passed, Clint sensed he needed to venture back west. He started his drive toward California, but it didn't feel right.

There was too much noise.

He drove instead to Arizona and stopped in Flagstaff.

He was back in nature, back in the quiet.

Still, the location wasn't quite right. He recalled a sign that stood out with the words "Sedona, AZ," and he drove there and pulled up into an RV park.

He was home.

WITH HIS BACKGROUND in stage lighting, Clint found a way to make ends meet. He wired the whole town with light art.

Then, one afternoon, a tour bus arrived. About 30-40 Japanese tourists filed out. They all had on white tennis shoes.

Although the sneaker stampede was a common occurrence, on this day Clint was different. The questions slammed right into him, "*Does it matter if we get disconnected from earth or if we're not grounded anymore? Does it affect us negatively?*"

The repetition of the white rubber soles hit home. The sneakers, the very shoes that protected people, also separated them from the ground.

Inspired, he rushed home to measure *grounded vs. not grounded*.

He used static and an EMF voltmeter on his body. He found that he returned to zero when he touched the grounded metal because it drew out his charge.

He took the inspiration further and placed the prepared metal on his bed.

Sleep came to him instantly that night. The earth connection completely changed the health of his body.

Joyfully, the higher power that had spoken to him and supported his journey brought him to an amazing realization—his mission in life. Clint set out to help others learn about his discovery, heal the world, and bring humanity back to nature.

THE PRACTICE

One of Clint's first-ever studies utilized a partnership with students at UCLA. Together they designed the study that supported a group of sixty people: thirty test subjects who practiced grounding for thirty days created the active group, and an equal number of test subjects who did not practice grounding for those days created the placebo group.

At the end of the study, the participants who practiced grounding had made significant changes. Some of these areas of change were TMJ and pain. One very vocal study member, a young girl in her early twenties, had excruciating menstrual cramps that forced her to take off work for the entire week of her period due to the pain. Halfway through the study, she couldn't believe it—she didn't have any cramps.

As TIME PASSED, Clint encountered many people with Lupus, MS, and Fibromyalgia, all of which are inflammation-related health issues, and all were helped by his Earthing methods.

For more than twenty years, Clint assisted doctors and advised them on the benefits of Earthing and how to use it, further expanding the impact of this natural healing method.

From his studies and experiences, he learned that men and women handle stress and life differently. Women are frequently more stressed. Because of this, 99% of women aged 30-55 have an inflammation-related health challenge. These challenges tend to increase physical, emotional, and mental pain to intolerable levels.

When pain is chronic, it reaches into every aspect of your life. For many, the loss of health is the loss of everything.

To avoid these losses, it is essential to discharge the cause of the inflammation and put out the fire. As soon as you get grounded, you release energy, and your pain calms. Your immune system returns to work and takes care of normal, necessary functions. Over time, a grounded individual's health returns.

With over 30 studies completed over 20 years, Clint validates the claim, "You cannot have inflammation in a grounded body." Thanks to his mission, over one million people know how easy it is to ground.

All you need is contact with the Earth!

Clint still encourages everyone to spend time outside in nature, connecting with the Earth. Whether you connect by walking barefoot on grass or sand, sitting on the ground, or using an Earthing product like a mat or sheet indoors, grounding is easy.

As Clint often shares, "What are you waiting for? Get out there and start grounding! Your body will thank you for it."[1]

---

1. Research References

    5. Electric Nutrition: The Surprising Health and Healing Benefits of Biological Grounding (Earthing).
    https://pubmed.ncbi.nlm.nih.gov/28987038/

    9. Classification of EEG Signal for Body Earthing Application 2018
    https://earthinginstitute.net/wp-content/uploads/2021/10/RahmanAl.EEG_for_Body-Earthing_Application-2018-1.pdf

    14. One-Hour Contact with the Earth's Surface (Grounding) Improves Inflammation and Blood Flow—A Randomized, Double-Blind, Pilot Study 2015
    www.scirp.org/Journal/PaperInformation.aspx?PaperID=58836

    15The Effect of Grounding the Human Body on Mood 2015
    prx.sagepub.com/content/116/2/534.full.pdf+html

    22. Emotional Stress, Heart Rate Variability, Grounding, and Improved Autonomic Tone: Clinical Applications 2011
    https://earthinginstitute.net/wp-content/uploads/2016/07/Emotional-stress-study.pdf

    30. The Biologic Effects of Grounding the Human Body During Sleep as Measured by Cortisol Levels and Subjective Reporting of Sleep, Pain, and Stress 2004
    https://earthinginstitute.net/wp-content/uploads/2016/07/Cortisol-Study.pdf

    42. Earthing: health implications of reconnecting the human body to the Earth's surface electrons.
    https://pubmed.ncbi.nlm.nih.gov/22291721/

    46. The effect of grounding the human body on mood.
    https://pubmed.ncbi.nlm.nih.gov/25748085/

    52. The biologic effects of grounding the human body during sleep as measured by cortisol levels and subjective reporting of sleep, pain, and stress.
    https://pubmed.ncbi.nlm.nih.gov/15650465/

AFTERWORD

THE MOTHER EARTH EFFECT, BOOK 2

It is with great anticipation that Elisabeth and Olivia ask you, the reader, to share your story.

Please send details of your journey with Earthing and grounding, how the process, methods, and products impact your life and the life of those you love, before and after images, and more to
themothereartheffect@gmail.com
or visit the site **https://www. themothereartheffect.com**

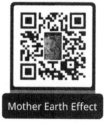

TheMotherEarthEffect.com

ACKNOWLEDGMENTS

We want to take this opportunity to acknowledge and thank the brave women who contributed these beautiful healing journeys to *Mother Earth Effect*. Their profound stories will surely inspire others dealing with the same or similar ailments. We recognize their strength and ability to overcome and conquer such debilitating conditions. We honor their soul connection, which allows them to vulnerably tell the world about the pain of their experience.

With our deepest gratitude, thank you.

We wish to express our profound appreciation to Clinton Ober, the man who rediscovered earthing. This endeavor would not have been possible without your helping hand guiding us through this project all the way to the end. Thank you for putting endless time and energy into this incredibly important initiative. With your support, we will achieve our goal of grounding more than 1 million women across the world.

ELISABETH HOEKSTRA

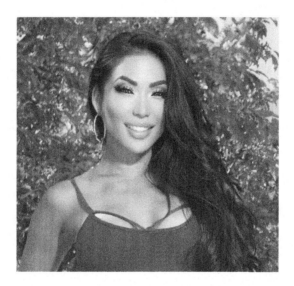

Elisabeth Hoekstra's first career was in the entertainment industry, where she worked as a model and actor on nationally syndicated television programs, movies, music videos, and magazines.

Elisabeth's evolution as an on-camera talent continued to expand while attending Davenport College for business management and marketing administration.

She returned to school in 2016 at Schoolcraft College, where she received her baking and pastry certification and mastered the art as a sous chef serving under one of the top pastry chefs in the country. Elisabeth worked at several prestigious venues during her culinary run including Oakland Hills Country Club, and she helped open and operate an award-winning restaurant, Otus Supply, in 2017.

Continuing to expand her entrepreneurial skills, Elisabeth received her real estate license in 2017. In 2018 she was named the exclusive real estate agent for a statewide campaign, during which she broke all records for securing the most offices in the briefest time. Elisabeth has also contributed significantly to nonprofits, focusing on children's health and education through hosting fundraisers and advocacy.

Throughout her various careers, she has seen how stress can take its toll on people's mental and physical well-being, leading her to work at a holistic wellness center. There, she quickly became company President, applying her knowledge in business and connections from previous careers.

This led to her current position as Director of Operations for the worldwide brand and TV network, 4biddenknowledge Inc. She is now helping to organize and grow 4biddenknowledge Inc. mainstream, all while hosting her popular podcast "Bio-Hack Your Best Life" alongside President/CEO of 4biddenknowledge, Billy Carson. Elisabeth's most recent accomplishments have been writing her first book, "The Recipe to Elevated Consciousness" which quickly became a best seller, as well as receiving a certificate in cell biology – mitochondria from Harvard University.

Currently, she's enrolled in the Neuroscience program at Harvard University.

Scan the QR-Code with your smartphone's camera or use the links to Follow Elisabeth

https://www.instagram.com/elisabethihoekstra/

https://www.facebook.com/iamelisabethhoekstra/

https://www.elisabethihoekstra.com/

https://www.tiktok.com/@elisabethihoekstra/

OLIVIA RAMIREZ SMITH

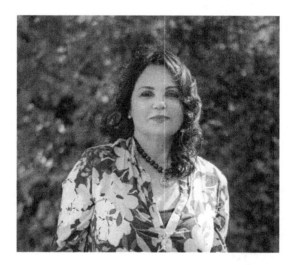

Olivia Smith is a co-producer of the award-winning Earthing Movie and well known as the Earthing ambassador, she is also a Master NLP Practitioner, Master Hypnotherapy Practitioner, and co-author of Sacred Spaces.

She developed her passion for supporting and empowering women while owning and operating a wellness center and spa for 17 years.

Above all, Olivia is an advocate for women's empowerment. For years, she has put women and the importance of their mental and emotional well-being at the forefront of her mind, and it quickly became her driving force. Over several years while producing the

Earthing Movie, Olivia began to identify what she feels is her true calling; teaching women about the significant mental and physical health benefits of Nature and Earthing.

Olivia also specializes in MER, the mental and emotional release technique, to release unresolved negative emotions and beliefs that hold us back from what we truly desire. As an Ambassador for Earthing, Olivia worked with The Chopra Center in assisting attendees in experiencing the benefits of grounding.

With Earthing alone serving as a powerful method to reduce stress, tension, and pain in the body, Olivia became a Master NLP Practitioner and a Master Hypnotherapy Practitioner to strengthen her ability to help women experience a more powerful and complete transformation.

Educating women about the necessity of grounding their body and mind in Nature is her Mission.

In Olivia's free time, she enjoys Pilates classes, barefoot walks, and hiking with her little Yorkie, Bodhi. Connect with Olivia on social media.

Scan the QR-Code with your smartphone camera or use the links to Follow Olivia

https://www.instagram.com/olivia_smith201/

https://www.facebook.com/oliviaramirez smith/

MAKE A CONNECTION

Throughout their healing journey, ALL the women featured in this book found miraculous ways to help themselves and others.

We appreciate them, as we are sure you do.

Learn more about the women who appear in *The Mother Earth Effect, Connect to the earth and heal.* Each can be contacted individually or through the website https://www.themoth ereartheffect.com.

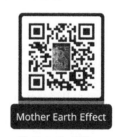

Mother Earth Effect

BRISA ALFARO   *TheMotherEarthEffect.com*

An International Speaker, Author, and Coach that captivates audiences with her powerful story of surviving a stroke with less than a one percent chance of recovery. Brisa achieved her miraculous recovery by making "Pinky Moves," consistent small actions that add up to life-changing results.

Brisa now works with individuals to unlock limitless possibilities, whether they are recovering from a stroke, or rising from a low point in life. She meets clients where they are and guides them to break out of their confining circumstances.

Whether appearing on national television, presenting to audiences all over the world, or working with private clients, Brisa shares her story and powerful "Pinky Moves" with honesty, humility, and grace.

You will love discovering how small moves can create BIG RESULTS.

Visit BrisaAlfaro.com or follow Brisa Alfaro on social media.

JENNIFER JOHNSON

A certified massage therapist, medical intuitive, and the Senior Director of Mind-Body Programs for Chopra Global working for over 19 years, Jennifer contributes as a core educator, creator, and master trainer. She loves to teach others how to improve their health, happiness, and healing using their innate intuitive response, connecting the mind-body.

Jennifer is passionate about energy medicine and somatic therapies as tools to identify the source of a person's disease or discomfort, ultimately leading to their unique expression of healing and wholeness.

Jennifer's singular mission is to help people find their joy by learning to connect to their bodies and shift their awareness. This shift, Jennifer teaches, supplies her clients with the knowledge they need to find their joy, better their lives, and spread happiness to those around them.

TAYA CRAYK-BONDE

A 29-year-old full-time mother and personal assistant, Taya has dabbled in many professions. The one she has enjoyed the most is creating art through writing, painting, and graphic design. She contributed the art for the cover of this wonderful book as well as The Mother Earth poem *Our One True Home* found at the beginning of the book.

Taya lives in sunny California with her fiancé Slater, her beautiful two-year-old daughter, Ember Skye, and her group of rambunctious but beloved pets. When she's not working, Taya loves to be in nature as much as she can, soaking in the beauty each day holds. Spending quality time with loved ones, creating art, playing outside with Ember, hiking, and exploring with her family.

If you are looking to connect or ask questions, Taya can be reached at taya.craykbonde@gmail.com. She can also be contacted via Facebook or Instagram under Taya Starr.

ASHLIE FLOOD

Ashlie is a natural health and rewilding enthusiast. In 2007, Ashlie took over accountability for her health and stopped relying on western ideologies for her well-being. By learning to care for her health and wellness intrinsically and from the perspective of the nervous system, she has become resilient and adaptive, free of disease, and in conscious co-creation with surrounding frequencies.

Using the connection to earth, movement, and community, she is now committed to helping others understand the power of working with the nervous system as a means of obtaining and maintaining health and happiness in life.

CHRISTINE CONTINI

In 2009, Christine was 38 years old and just getting her feet firmly back on the ground. While experiencing improved health for the first time in her life, Christine had the misfortune of suffering a massive heart attack and a near-death experience, which you can read about in her book *Death, Awakening to Life*.

While on the other side, Christine gathered vital information that can be used for the healing of our world. She spends her time as a writer, speaker, educator, mother, grandmother, and more.

Christine admits she is far too busy to update her social media but encourages you to enjoy her shares from the past on her website https://christinecontini.com/

PATRICIA HACKER

Patricia is an author, entrepreneur, and passionate environmental and health advocate. Most recently she has developed her own company, World Wellbeing, which focuses on projects and collaborations to heal and restore our physical world and all its inhabitants.

Patricia believes it is critical to provide people with foundational mental and physical well-being tools, services, and products to thrive in an ever-changing and increasingly challenging world. This support allows them to amplify their compassionate lifestyle choices required to drive climate change reversal.

SAMIA MCCULLY, ND

A licensed naturopathic doctor for 18 years, Samia is the owner and founder of Wellness Architecture—a boutique wellness clinic located in downtown Menlo Park, CA. Dr. McCully has helped thousands of high-performing women resolve fatigue and impossible weight loss, restoring the energy, vitality, and confidence they had in their younger years.

She has been heard on NPR, published many health-related articles, mentored students at the Stanford Graduate School of business, and taught at many other highly regarded institutions.

Her passion for travel and different cultures has led Samia to live in Korea, Abu Dhabi, Canada, and Lebanon. She currently lives with her husband and three kids in Menlo Park, California. Visit her at www.wellnessarchitecture.com

BILLIE RINEHART

Born in the country of Panama, Billie is a mother of two, an avid reader, and passionate about implementing different modalities to maintain a healthy lifestyle.

'Miss-Adventures' a recently launched book collaboration she was a part of became an Amazon Bestseller in 5 categories.

Billie has always been enthusiastic about elevating other women. For this reason, she holds Goddess Circles to create a space where women can gather to connect, release and enlighten their lives.

STACY PLAZIAK

At 56, Stacy is a five-year cancer survivor. She lives in Escondido California and has three amazing daughters. Stacy works as a sales manager for a mailbox company and enjoys working with people and building relationships.

In her spare time, she enjoys wine tasting, baseball games, walks on the beach with her dog, and spending time with family and friends. As a woman of faith, Stacy believes in paying it forward with gratitude.

TERESA PODGORSKI

A nationally certified physician assistant for 21 years, Teresa's area of practice is adult medicine. She graduated Magna Cum Laude from Charles R. Drew University of Science & Medicine in 2000, and also attended the University of California Riverside where she was a member of the Golden Key International Honor Society. Teresa attended Victor Valley College and was a member of the Phi Theta Kappa Honor Society.

An avid hiker, reader, and dog lover, Teresa has resided in the High Desert since 1989, except for 2 years while attending Drew.

JULIENNE DALLARA

An actor/singer/dancer who woke up paralyzed in 1996, Julienne's story is truly amazing. At the time that she was struck down with this rare disease, Transverse Myelitis, Julienne had her daughter, then 3 years old, and her son, 7 months, to care for. Being in a wheelchair was a challenge.

When her husband left, not able to deal with this impossible change in their lives, Julienne began a career selling accessible vehicles. Doing this, she met her husband of 20 years, another wheelchair user with post-polio.

In 2012, Julienne was approached by the Abilities Expo to be a salesperson for this vital chain of National trade shows that showcase products for people with disabilities. Working there is a joy; fulfilling her need to help others while still allowing her to exercise her passion for gardening and creating fine art.

GABRIELLE FORLEO

Money Mindset Maven + Business Mentor. Gabrielle helps women create a life and business that makes the money they desire with the freedom and ease they deserve. Chopra Total Wellbeing Certified + 16 years of Coaching + thousands of clients served around the world. Gabrielle is an expert at helping women become self-funded and self-trusted.

GET TO KNOW THE EARTHING PRODUCTS!

TRY SOME OF THE MANY EVERYDAY WAYS TO USE EARTHING PRODUCTS

YOUR FEET WILL THANK YOU

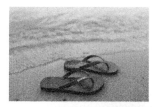

Don't let plastic-soled shoes get in the way of grounding. Grounders ground you when outside on grass, cement, sand, dirt, or gravel.

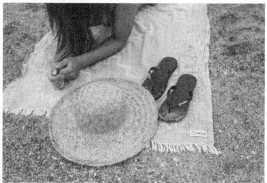

ENJOY BLISSFUL, GROUNDED SLEEP

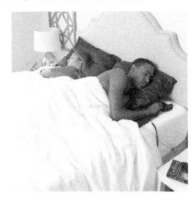

With no perforations in the surface of these Mattress Covers, they are more comfortable for sleeping while keeping you 100% grounded no matter where you move.

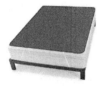

The hypoallergenic nature of the carbon material helps combat allergens in your bed. In addition to grounding, the sheet creates a bonus physical shield against the dust and mites living in your mattress.

The Earthing Elite™ Pillow Cover envelopes any regular-size pillow to easily ground you while you sleep.

themotherearteffect.com

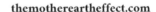

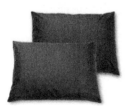

QUICK FIX BODY ISSUES

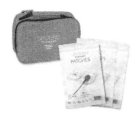

Patches can be used anywhere you stretch, work out, sit, relax, or sleep. Apply patches to any part of the body for targeted pain relief and reduction of inflammation or injury.

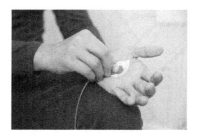

Patches can also be applied to the palms of the hands or the bottom of the feet as these are the most conductive points on the body.

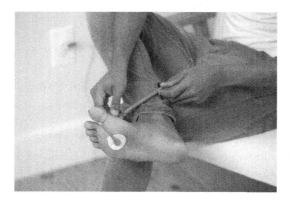

DAILY USE AROUND HOME

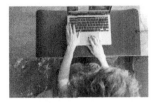

The Earthing Universal Mat is themothereartheffect.com's most versatile product! Use this mat on top of a desk under your keyboard and mouse, or under your desk to put your feet on. Put it on a couch to sit on, or on the back of the couch to lean against.

You can easily move your Universal Mat around your kitchen. Stand on the mat while washing dishes, prepping dinner, and cooking at the stove.

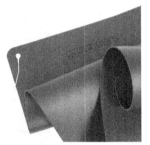

Keep the mat in your bedroom or bathroom for constant use for personal care.

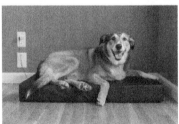

The Pet Bed Cover is naturally antimicrobial, fluid-resistant, and stain-resistant. This safe and durable cover grounds your pets while indoors.

The grounded Pet Bed Cover is a perfect car product with a smooth side for your pet to relax on, and a non-skid, self-ventilating mesh bottom. The entire cover is designed to withstand the normal wear and tear of indoor pets.

themothereartheffect.com

ENHANCE YOUR LIFE WITH
THEMOTHEREARTHEFFECT.COM

Every quality product you choose to enhance your earthing experience gives you constant grounded contact with Mother Earth.

Earth's natural energy stabilizes the way the body works at the deepest level, draining it of inflammation, pain, and stress, and generating greater well-being.

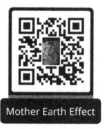

TheMotherEarthEffect.com

LINK INDEX

ARTICLES AND STUDIES

Throughout, you will see footnotes that share pertinent links to scientific information regarding the validity of grounding and Earthing Studies. The links listed are relevant to each personal experience in The Mother Earth Effect.

Links specific to a personal journey can be found in the footnotes of each chapter.

The Link Index is divided into three sections for your convenience:
   Earthing Studies
   Earthing Review Articles
   PubMed Studies
   At the time of printing, all links were found to be current. Titles of studies and articles are provided in the event that future links may change.

EARTHING STUDIES

1. Grounding the Body Improves Sleep Quality in Patients with Mild Alzheimer's Disease: A Pilot Study 2022
   https://www.ncbi.nlm.nih.gov/pmc/articles/PMC8954071/

2. How Localized Grounding, Combined with Conductive Skincare, Improves the Outcomes of the Traditional Skincare? 2021
   https://www.researchgate.net/publication/353156602_How_Localized_Grounding_Combined_with_Conductive_Skincare_Improves_the_Outcomes_of_the_Traditional_Skincare

3. A double-blind randomized trial to assess the efficacy of Jing Advanced Clinical Massage and Earthing as interventions in the treatment of chronic low back pain 2021
   https://begrounded.co.uk/earthing-research/

4. The Effects of Grounding on Meditation Quality: A Preliminary Study Report 2019 (abstract)
   https://earthinginstitute.net/the-effects-of-grounding-on-meditation-quality-a-preliminary-study-report/

5. Effectiveness of Grounded Sleeping on Recovery after Intensive Eccentric Muscle Loading 2019
https://www.frontiersin.org/articles/10.3389/fphys.2019.00035/full

6. The Effects of Grounding (Earthing) on Bodyworkers' Pain and Overall Quality of Life: A randomized Controlled Trial 2019
https://www.sciencedirect.com/science/article/pii/S1550830718302519

7. Grounding Patients With Hypertension Improves Blood Pressure: A Case History Series Study 2018
http://alternative-therapies.com/openaccess/26-6_Elkin.pdf

8. Effects of Grounding (Earthing) on Massage Therapists 2018
http://www.scirp.org/Journal/PaperInformation.aspx?PaperID=82706

9. Classification of EEG Signal for Body Earthing Application 2018
https://earthinginstitute.net/wp-content/uploads/2021/10/RahmanAl.EEG_for_Body-Earthing_Application-2018-1.pdf

10. Electrical Grounding Improves Vagal Tone in Preterm Infants 2017
https://www.karger.com/Article/Abstract/475744
View study charts here:
https://earthinginstitute.net/wp-content/uploads/2018/03/groundingprematurebabiesposter.pdf

11. Effects of Grounding on Body Voltage and Current in the Presence of Electromagnetic Fields 2016
https://earthinginstitute.net/wp-content/uploads/2016/06/Effects-of-Grounding-on-Body-Voltage-and-Current-in-the-Presence-of-Electromagnetic-Fields-2016.pdf

12. Health Effects of Alkaline Diet and Water, Reduction of Digestive-tract Bacterial Load, and Earthing 2016

https://www.academia.edu/33495468/Health_Effects_of_Alka line_Diet_and_Water_Reduction_of_Digestive_tract_Bacterial_Load _and_Earthing?auto=download&email_work_card=download-paper

13. Grounding After Moderate Eccentric Contractions Reduces Muscle Damage 2015

https://www.dovepress.com/articles.php?article_id=23771

14. One-Hour Contact with the Earth's Surface (Grounding) Improves Inflammation and Blood Flow—A Randomized, Double-Blind, Pilot Study 2015

http://www.scirp.org/Journal/PaperInformation.aspx?PaperID= 58836

15. The Effect of Grounding the Human Body on Mood 2015

http://prx.sagepub.com/content/116/2/534.full.pdf+html

16. Grounding the Human Body during Yoga Exercise with a Grounded Yoga Mat Reduces Blood Viscosity 2015

http://www.scirp.org/Journal/PaperInformation.aspx?PaperID= 55445#.VSa19_nF_7A

17. An Experimental Study on Immediate Effect of Direct Barefoot Contact with Earth on Prehypertension 2015

https://earthinginstitute.net/wp-content/uploads/2021/03/Shiv ayogappaAl.-Immediate-effects-of-barefoot-contact-with-eath-on-prehypertension-2015.pdf

18. Grounding the Human Body Improves Facial Blood Flow Regulation 2014

http://www.scirp.org/journal/PaperInformation.aspx?PaperID= 51326#.VHDemfnF8SA

19. Differences in Blood Urea and Creatinine Concentrations in Earthed and Unearthed Subjects during Cycling Exercise and Recovery 2013
   http://www.hindawi.com/journals/ecam/2013/382643/

20. Earthing (Grounding) the Human Body Reduces Blood Viscosity —a Major Factor in Cardiovascular Disease 2013Additionally,
   http://online.liebertpub.com/doi/pdfplus/10.1089/acm.
2011.0820
   to view the Blood Viscosity Video Clip click here:
   https://earthinginstitute.net/how-grounding-affects-blood-viscosity/

21. Earthing the Human Organism Influences Bioelectrical Processes 2012
   https://earthinginstitute.net/wp-content/uploads/2016/07/Sokal-and-Sokal-2012-Bioelectrical-processes.pdf

22. Emotional Stress, Heart Rate Variability, Grounding, and Improved Autonomic Tone: Clinical Applications 2011
   https://earthinginstitute.net/wp-content/uploads/2016/07/Emotional-stress-study.pdf

23. Earthing the Human Body Influences Physiologic Processes 2011. Editorial: Chronic Disease: Are We Missing Something?
   https://www.ncbi.nlm.nih.gov/pmc/articles/PMC3154031/
   https://earthinginstitute.net/wp-content/uploads/2019/12/Oschmaneditorial-2011-1.pdf

24. Pilot Study on the Effect of Grounding on Delayed-Onset Muscle Soreness 2010
   https://earthinginstitute.net/wp-content/uploads/2016/11/Brown_Chevalier_Hill_earthing_delayed_muscle_2010.pdf

25. Earthing effects in Lewis Rats 2010

https://earthinginstitute.net/wp-content/uploads/2021/03/Earth
ing-effects-in-Lewis-Rats-2010.pdf

26. Changes in Pulse Rate, Respiratory Rate, Blood Oxygenation, Perfusion Index, Skin Conductance, and Their Variability Induced During and After Grounding Human Subjects for 40 Minutes 2010
    https://earthinginstitute.net/wp-content/uploads/2016/07/
Changes-in-Pulse-Rate-Study.pdf

27. The Effect Of Earthing On Human Physiology, Part 2 2007
    http://journals.sfu.ca/seemj/index.php/seemj/article/view/9/7

28. The Effect Of Earthing On Human Physiology, Part 1 2006
    https://earthinginstitute.net/wp-content/uploads/2019/12/
Effect-of-Earthing-on-Human-Physiology-Part-1.pdf

29. The Effectiveness of a Conductive Patch and a Conductive Bed Pad in Reducing Induced Human Body Voltage Via the Application of Earth Ground 2005
    https://earthinginstitute.net/wp-content/uploads/2019/12/Apple
white-Body-Voltage-study.pdf

30. The Biologic Effects of Grounding the Human Body During Sleep as Measured by Cortisol Levels and Subjective Reporting of Sleep, Pain, and Stress 2004
    https://earthinginstitute.net/wp-content/uploads/2016/07/Corti
sol-Study.pdf

31. Thermography Case Histories 2004-2005
    https://earthinginstitute.net/wp-content/uploads/2019/02/
thermographycasehistories2004.pdf

32. Initial Grounding Experimentation by Clint Ober, 2000 (as part of a brief historical review of Earthing)
    https://earthinginstitute.net/brief-history-of-earthing/

EARTHING REVIEW ARTICLES

33. Integrative and Lifestyle Medicine Strategies Should Include Earthing (Grounding): Review of Research Evidence and Clinical Observations 2020
    https://www.sciencedirect.com/science/article/pii/S1550830719305476

34. Electric Nutrition: The Surprising Health and Healing Benefits of Biological Grounding (Earthing)Altern Ther Health Med.
    http://www.alternative-therapies.com/index.cfm/fuseaction/Content.Main/id/2123/OA-ElectricNutrition:TheSurprisingHealthandHealingBenefitsofBiologicalGrounding(Earthing)
    https://www.ncbi.nlm.nih.gov/pubmed/28987038

35. Prevention and Treatment of Influenza, Influenza-Like Illness, and Common Clod by Herbal, Complementary, and Natural Therapies 2017
    https://www.ncbi.nlm.nih.gov/pmc/articles/PMC5871211/

36. The Effects of Grounding (Earthing) on Inflammation, Immune Response, Wound Healing, and Prevention and Treatment of Chronic Inflammatory and Autoimmune Diseases 2015
    https://www.dovepress.com/articles.php?article_id=21001

37. Biophysics of Earthing (grounding) the Human Body, in Bioelectromagnetic and Subtle Energy Medicine (CRC Press), 2015
    https://earthinginstitute.net/wp-content/uploads/2018/05/biophysics-of-earthing-grounding-the-human-body-2015.pdf

38. Health Implications of Reconnecting the Human Body to the Earth's Surface Electrons 2012
    http://www.hindawi.com/journals/jeph/2012/291541/

39. The Neuromodulative Role of Earthing 2011
    http://www.medical-hypotheses.com/article/S0306-9877(11)00364-1/abstract

PUBMED STUDIES

PubMed is a free resource supporting the search and retrieval of biomedical and life sciences literature with the aim of improving health–both globally and personally.

40. Integrative and lifestyle medicine strategies should include Earthing (grounding):
    Review of research evidence and clinical observations.
    https://pubmed.ncbi.nlm.nih.gov/31831261/

41. The effects of grounding (earthing) on inflammation, the immune response, wound healing, and prevention and treatment of chronic inflammatory and autoimmune diseases.
    https://pubmed.ncbi.nlm.nih.gov/25848315/

42. Earthing: health implications of reconnecting the human body to the Earth's surface electrons.
    https://pubmed.ncbi.nlm.nih.gov/22291721/

43. The Effects of Grounding (Earthing) on Bodyworkers' Pain and Overall Quality of Life: A Randomized Controlled Trial.

https://pubmed.ncbi.nlm.nih.gov/30448083/

44. Electric Nutrition: The Surprising Health and Healing Benefits of Biological Grounding (Earthing).
   https://pubmed.ncbi.nlm.nih.gov/28987038/

45. Earthing (grounding) the human body reduces blood viscosity-a major factor in cardiovascular disease.
   https://pubmed.ncbi.nlm.nih.gov/22757749/

46. The effect of grounding the human body on mood.
   https://pubmed.ncbi.nlm.nih.gov/25748085/

47. Prevention and treatment of COVID-19 infection by earthing.
   https://pubmed.ncbi.nlm.nih.gov/35987499/

48. Grounding after moderate eccentric contractions reduces muscle damage.
   https://pubmed.ncbi.nlm.nih.gov/26443876/

49. Grounding Patients With Hypertension Improves Blood Pressure: A Case History Series Study.
   https://pubmed.ncbi.nlm.nih.gov/30982019/

50. Can electrons act as antioxidants? A review and commentary.
   https://pubmed.ncbi.nlm.nih.gov/18047442/

51. Charge transfer in the living matrix.
   https://pubmed.ncbi.nlm.nih.gov/19524846/

52. The biologic effects of grounding the human body during sleep as measured by cortisol levels and subjective reporting of sleep, pain, and stress.
   https://pubmed.ncbi.nlm.nih.gov/15650465/

53. The Impact of Grounding in Running Shoes on Indices of Performance in Elite Competitive Athletes.
   https://pubmed.ncbi.nlm.nih.gov/35162340/

54. Analysis of the charge exchange between the human body and ground: evaluation of "earthing" from an electrical perspective.
   https://pubmed.ncbi.nlm.nih.gov/25435837/

—